YOGA OF RECOVERY

of related interest

Yoga Therapy for Fear
Treating Anxiety, Depression and Rage with the Vagus Nerve and Other Techniques
Beth Spindler
ISBN 978 1 84819 374 1
eISBN 978 0 85701 331 6

Yoga for Grief and Loss
Poses, Meditation, Devotion, Self-Reflection, Selfless Acts, Ritual
Karla Helbert
Foreword by Chinnamasta Stiles
ISBN 978 1 84819 204 1
eISBN 978 0 85701 163 3

The Chakras in Grief and Trauma
A Tantric Guide to Energetic Wholeness
Karla Helbert
Illustrated by Rachel Rosenkoetter
ISBN 978 1 84819 365 9
eISBN 978 0 85701 324 8

Teen Yoga for Yoga Therapists
A Guide to Development, Mental Health and Working with Common Teen Issues
Charlotta Martinus
Foreword by Sir Anthony Seldon
ISBN 978 1 84819 399 4
eISBN 978 0 85701 355 2

YOGA OF RECOVERY

Integrating Yoga and Ayurveda with Modern Recovery Tools for Addiction

DURGA LEELA

Foreword by David Frawley

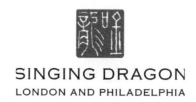

SINGING DRAGON
LONDON AND PHILADELPHIA

First published in Great Britain in 2022 by Singing Dragon,
an imprint of Jessica Kingsley Publishers
An imprint of Hodder & Stoughton Ltd
An Hachette Company

2

Copyright © Durga Leela 2022
Foreword © David Frawley 2022

The information contained in this book is not intended to replace the services of trained medical professionals or to be a substitute for medical advice. The complementary therapy described in this book may not be suitable for everyone to follow. You are advised to consult a doctor before embarking on any complementary therapy program and on any matters relating to your health, and in particular on any matters that may require diagnosis or medical attention.

A CIP catalogue record for this title is available from the
British Library and the Library of Congress

ISBN 978 1 78775 755 4
eISBN 978 1 78775 756 1

Printed and bound in Great Britain by CPI Group

Jessica Kingsley Publishers' policy is to use papers that are natural, renewable and recyclable products and made from wood grown in sustainable forests. The logging and manufacturing processes are expected to conform to the environmental regulations of the country of origin.

Jessica Kingsley Publishers
Carmelite House
50 Victoria Embankment
London EC4Y 0DZ

www.singingdragon.com

Contents

Acknowledgments

Every step of this journey has been guided by community, inspired by teachers and mentors. I offer great gratitude to David Frawley whose many books have guided me and whose words you will find abundantly in this book. I thank Swami Sitaramananda, Swami Swaroopananda, Swami Karunananda and all the staff at the Sivananda and Integral Yoga ashrams and centers for hosting Yoga of Recovery since 2005. I thank Dr. Claudia Welch, Dr. Ramkumar Kutty and Dr. Robert Svoboda who have all contributed greatly through their teaching, articles and books. I am grateful to Richard Miller and his team for the years of work they have done to get iRest approved as a complementary and alternative medicine warranting continuing research for its use in the treatment of PTSD and as a Tier 1 approach for addressing pain management in military care.

Other supporters are Michele Lawrence (Inner Peace Yoga Therapy), Monique Lonner (Soul of Yoga), Tommy Rosen (Recovery 2.0), Phil Valentine (CCAR), Jivana Heyman (Accessible Yoga), Amanda Ree (Chopra Center and now Sama Dog), Nirmala Raniga (Chopra Addiction and Wellness Center), Sarahjoy Marsh (Daya Foundation), Felicia Tomasko (LA Yoga and Ayurveda) and Abby (Abhaya) Geyer (NAMA and IAYT) and Nikky Myers (Y12SR). Thank you for championing the Yoga of Recovery conversation within your offerings. Deep gratitude and love to all the YoR assistants over the years, I could not have done this without your support.

Thank you Grace Welker for helping me form the structure and words of this book. Thanks to Tarini (Shanna Ramakrishnan) for coaxing me to show up on social media. And finally thanks to my family, friends, sponsors and especially my husband Vanasiva/Josh, for sticking by me through all these years.

I offer my sincere thanks to the people who truly make Yoga of Recovery—everyone who has come to YoR retreats and courses over the years, and everyone we are yet to meet. You are all very special to me. I am honored to be in a healing circle with you and hope this book will help widen our circle so we can stick together and continue to heal the heartache addiction causes.

FOREWORD

Addiction has become one of the world's main health problems at both a physical and psychological level: it affects young and old alike and is reaching epidemic proportions, including in the USA. There are many types, from sugar and food to alcohol, recreational and pharmaceutical drugs, as well as behavioral and media addictions.

The question is not only how to treat addiction at a chemical level—which has been widely explored—but also how to treat it at the more fundamental behavioral, mind and consciousness levels. New insights are clearly needed to broaden the basis of treatment and help those in recovery from falling back into old patterns. This is where Yoga and related Ayurvedic approaches are helpful, as they offer a new, transformative view of self-awareness to counter compulsions.

According to Yoga, the mind tends toward addiction. Part of this is simply because our behavior is habitual and conditioned, based upon external stimuli that we can easily become attached to. We compulsively go after what affords us pleasure or distraction, or gives us a state of inebriation, in which our problems can temporarily be forgotten.

Yoga and Ayurvedic practitioners commonly come into contact with clients who suffer from addiction at various levels. *Yoga of Recovery* provides them the special insight and practices they can share to address this increasing problem in a fundamental manner. While several books have addressed the problem of addiction through discussions of Yogic ideas and the relevance of meditation, this book is perhaps the most specific and in depth, and brings in Ayurveda in a primary and detailed manner.

Durga Leela experienced a life-threatening addiction and discovered how to use Yoga and Ayurveda to recover.

She began teaching others how to do the same, and has now taught worldwide for many years with the renowned Sivananda Yoga organization. She brings a rare experience of treating addiction at both a personal level and as a trained Yoga teacher. Her book has a deep spiritual perspective, but also offers a practical approach that can be adopted by anyone.

As someone who has taught Yoga and Ayurveda for several decades and also knows Durga and has discussed these topics with her, I am happy to endorse her approach and hope that everyone working in the field of addiction, especially with a respect for Yoga and Ayurveda, will examine this book carefully.

According to Yoga philosophy, happiness and bliss is our original divine nature. But to experience it we must learn how to calm the mind and live in harmony with our unique constitution, as guided by a spiritual aspiration. To achieve this, Yoga, Ayurveda and meditation are essential. May this inspiring book help its readers reclaim that inner happiness and learn how to counter the addictive tendencies of the mind as part of total well-being!

David Frawley, author of Ayurveda and the Mind *and* Yoga and Ayurveda
director at the American Institute of Vedic Studies

INTRODUCTION

OUR UNDERSTANDING OF OUR SUFFERING defines the nature of our solution.[1] My own path in founding Yoga of Recovery (YoR) stems from being a child of an alcoholic, becoming alcoholic myself in my teens, finding Yoga in my mid-20s, a few suicide attempts and losing my mother to alcoholism when I was 32 years old. Shortly after that, I was fired from a job I was headhunted into. Then I "did a geographic"—moving from London to Lake Tahoe to take a year off and sort myself out, but wherever you go, there you are, and after nine months in the USA, my new life was in shambles. I once again felt desperate, but this time I took myself to a meeting of AA (Alcoholics Anonymous) and experienced almost instant relief from my obsession with alcohol. What made the transformative experience of sobriety a sustainable, ongoing process was the "blossoming" of that foundation of sobriety, service and fellowship (the three pillars of 12-Step principles) to a life of balance through Ayurveda and a life of purpose through Yoga. These three modalities are available to me in every moment of my life in the small everyday choices and larger life decisions, and now I'm honored to have the opportunity to share this here with you.

YoR integrates the wisdom of Yoga and Ayurveda with modern recovery tools. It is open to all who are looking to overcome self-destructive or addictive tendencies. This powerful combination offers us a truly empowering way to *embody* a personal program of recovery.

YoR offers a unique perspective and presentation of Ayurveda. The topics selected from this vast system of knowledge are chosen to make Ayurveda instantly relatable, accessible and current for people in recovery, to help shift their life trajectory. I truly believe Ayurveda is the best system of behavioral health care for all modern chronic diseases. The toolbox is full and many are thankful that Ayurveda offers these tools and suggestions beyond the usual diet and exercise dogma we've been offered for years from the health and fitness industry. Ayurveda offers general advice for all of us; YoR presents this information in a way that allows the person to draw out what will help them most at their particular point of the recovery path—which is a lifetime journey.

Ayurveda is a humanistic and person-centered medicine. Addiction is a serious social plague that takes many forms in our modern-day society (bio-psycho-social-emotional-spiritual-cultural-economic-political etc.). It is a disease of spirit, mind and body and for that we need an understanding of ourselves at each of these levels, and also an understanding of the disease in each aspect of our being so we can live the solution. This is important as we not only see the misery of addiction spread through the many widely available substances and addictive behaviors, but also how it adversely affects all those whose lives are touched by it.

So here is the science of life, the science of self-healing to help all of us to reconnect with our earlier innocence and brightness. You can make use of any part of this book at any stage of your addiction experience. This is not exclusively aimed at the person with substance use disorder, in the early stages of recovery, as most of the money, attention and efforts of the disease-based medical model have focused on the acute care model. It really is time to add a holistic continuum of care.

Yoga of Recovery is for people who are looking to overcome any of their own addictive or self-destructive behaviors and also for people with histories of addiction in themselves or within their family. This book is also for Yoga teachers, Yoga therapists and addiction counselors/coaches who are working with people suffering from addiction. YoR guests have ranged from 16 to 84 years old and experience every type of addiction—this means both the "primary" addiction and all the cross-addictions that have come up since abstaining from the "substance/behavior of choice." We look at common stress responses, unmanaged emotions, how the mind works by repetition, leading to deep grooves of self-destructive habits.

YoR's treatment method follows a diagnosis that reflects the Yogic system of medicine and its theory of disease. Ayurveda treats disease and teaches principles for right living. It is a complete Yogic system of medicine.

This book helps us understand the areas in which people may become vulnerable when under stress—and determine what kinds of activities and changes in lifestyle can best help restore balance in mind and body. The aim is to revitalize the body/mind system so we have a strong foundation in health to face the challenges and stresses of daily life without resorting/relapsing into old addictive behaviors.

YoR incorporates the sister sciences of Yoga and Ayurveda and offers ways to become free from our self-defeating lifestyles. It helps us to *embody* our recovery. Here you'll learn methods for utilizing the principles and practices of Ayurveda and Yoga to heal the root causes of chronic diseases, psychological problems, addictions and eating disorders.

ENDNOTE

1   Gates, R. & Kenison, K. (2002) *Meditations from the Mat: Daily Reflections on the Path of Yoga*. New York: Anchor Books, pp. 108–109.

Chapter 1

THE ROOT OF ALL DISEASE IS SPIRITUAL

THE LAST STRAW

I WENT TO A YOGA ASHRAM in 2001 in a bid to stop smoking. It happened because of a challenge from my therapist, who had suggested I see a psychiatrist who diagnosed me as clinically depressed and prescribed antidepressants. I was wary of being medicated. I was still using nicotine (15–20 cigarettes per day) and now I was being advised to medicate to help my mood and mind. I was 18 months abstinent from alcohol at this time. The therapist suggested that I start by cutting one cigarette out per day with the goal of becoming a non-smoker at the end of two weeks. The first week was easy; the second was torture. Giving up alcohol seemed easier than giving up cigarettes.

Then, on day 11 of my nicotine rehabilitation experiment/"trying to stop smoking" period, I attended a party hosted by my AA sponsor. I was so on edge with my effort to stop smoking that my body physically ached with the tension. At the party, a woman suggested that I go to an ashram (a place for practicing Yoga, meditation and other spiritual practices to evolve and grow spiritually) as a supportive way to get through the initial days of abstinence. At the ashram, smoking is not allowed and the structured daily schedule with practices of Yoga and breathing exercises would help me connect in a healthy, more conscious way to my body. At this point, I was willing to try anything as I was reluctant to get out of bed and was sleeping ten hours at night, plus naps just to get through the day. I needed support.

All through this, I was aware of the insanity. I would look at the individual cigarette and wonder how such a small, insignificant item could somehow dominate and take over all my intelligence, reason and logic. To watch the effect this "trying to stop" was having on my mind was incredible. How could an intelligent human succumb to this inanimate object, letting it run her life— ruin her life!—taking away all pleasure and joy, creating a ceaseless stream of thoughts about how I would fail, how I could not get through one day without a cigarette, how I needed to be sequestered from society in order to achieve complete abstinence, and even then beware anyone who encountered me in this craving state. I was irritable, emotional, impatient—unable to live with myself if I made a decision to continue to be a smoker, but seemingly unable to become a non-smoker. Did I mention that I have asthma? All this mental anguish was accompanied by the regular need to take blasts on an inhaler, just to keep the wheezing at bay.

I loved cigarettes, they were my "friends," I was a committed smoker but I was also an alcoholic in recovery with over a year sober and I knew that smoking cigarettes was an ongoing addiction that was killing me. I did feel depressed. In the back of my mind, I also knew that I had unrealistic expectations about the antidepressants they were planning to give me. I was looking for the "Happy Pill" and would be disappointed with anything less. I had a sneaking suspicion that antidepressants would not meet my expectations of chemically induced happiness so this thought also came up often to sabotage my efforts at quitting.

On the day I was supposed to be on zero cigarettes, I sat on my deck completely and utterly defeated, tears streaming down my face; I quietly sobbed as I gazed at the full moon in the sky. I begged my Higher Power to remove my obsession with cigarettes. My prayer was answered and the next day I had been relieved of my nicotine obsession. That was over 20 years ago.

A few days after this incredible shift, I did go to the ashram to support my recovery. And it would change my life. Not only was I nicotine-free, I began learning the life-promoting practices of classical Yoga and Ayurveda.

REGAINING BALANCE

After my first visit to the ashram, I returned within one month. Both Ayurveda and Yoga felt so true, real and useful; I was excited to study more. It felt so good to visit the ashram, I even decided I'd take the Yoga Teachers Training

Course scheduled for the following year, mainly as a personal challenge and investment in my own sense of well-being. I was still struggling with a host of bothersome health issues like constipation, asthmatic breathing issues and extremely painful monthly periods due to endometriosis, and I felt lucky to have found this place to restore my health.

I'd leave the ashram with a feeling of empowerment—but within just a few days back at home I'd lapse back into an irregular lifestyle, exhausted by the work I was doing in therapy: processing hurts around friends/boyfriends, feeling hopeless regarding my sister's alcoholism and mental illness. There were so many emotions, and I felt sad, lonely, hurt, abandoned, angry, depressed. I knew I used my inappropriate boyfriend like a drug, I didn't exercise, ate too much and berated myself for being lazy and not getting anything accomplished.

This was peppered with feelings of such gratitude that I lived in Lake Tahoe and had found Ayurveda. My low days were interspersed with times where I felt more and more happy, whole and self-contained. Being sober and a non-smoker made life feel really good. I'd swing between these feeling states within any one week, sometimes in any one day.

Through all these highs and lows, there was something that was truly offering me hope. During my second visit to the ashram I'd heard Dr. Marc Halpern (founder of the California College of Ayurveda, CCA) give a talk on Ayurveda. He said that this ancient science of healing explained that disease begins when we forget our true nature as spirit, when we forget that the Universal Intelligence/divinity resides within each of us.

In other words, if we understand ourselves only as body and mind, we become overly identified and limited by the nature of the physical world. This was very interesting to me as it fit with what I'd been told in AA: that addiction was a "spiritual malady" and that I was "spiritually sick."[1] The *Big Book of Alcoholics Anonymous* (the primary text of the program of Alcoholics Anonymous) says that we are "beyond human aid"[2]—"Our human resources, as marshaled by the will, were not sufficient: they failed utterly."[3] I had never considered that prospect/explanation before entering AA but when I heard it there, it made sense to me; the more efforts I made to marshal my will and stop drinking and smoking, the more I felt an utter failure, never being able to manage what I set out to do. And now I saw that this ancient healing science of Ayurveda was saying the same thing.

PERSPECTIVES ON THE DISEASE OF ADDICTION

Ayurveda views not only addiction as a spiritual malady but all disease; it is an all-encompassing diagnosis for the human race. We are here because we have forgotten our spiritual origins, we are ignorant of our true nature.

Table 1.1 shows a comparison of what Ayurveda, Yoga, the 12-Step programs and the Western model say about addiction.

Table 1.1 What Ayurveda, Yoga, the 12-Step programs and the Western model say about addiction

Ayurveda	The primordial cause of all disease is forgetting your true nature is spirit.
Yoga	All disease is a form of spiritual ignorance (Avidya).
12-Step programs	Alcoholism (addiction) is a "spiritual malady."[4]
National Institute on Drug Abuse (NIDA) currently subscribes to the brain disease model of addiction (BDMA)	"Addiction is defined as a chronic, relapsing brain disease that is characterized by compulsive drug seeking and use, despite harmful consequences. It is considered a brain disease because drugs change the brain—they change its structure and how it works. These brain changes can be long lasting, and can lead to the harmful behaviors seen in people who abuse drugs. Often require repeated treatments, and require a level of continuous care or support in order to be successful."[5] This has now been reworded to the following: "Addiction is defined as a chronic, relapsing disorder characterized by compulsive drug seeking, continued use despite harmful consequences, and long-lasting changes in the brain. It is considered both a complex brain disorder and a mental illness. Addiction is the most severe form of a full spectrum of substance use disorders, and is a medical illness caused by repeated misuse of a substance or substances."[6]

I had recovered from alcoholism and drug use through the spiritual program of the 12 Steps adhering to this advice: "What we really have is a daily reprieve contingent on the maintenance of our spiritual condition."[7] Now I was finding greater hope, empowerment and personal vitality from the addition of the spiritually based understanding of disease offered by both Ayurveda and Yoga. I discovered that Ayurveda offered a similar perspective on the suffering of addiction, but not only addictions—Ayurveda held this view for all disease. This talk about the Ayurveda root cause of disease was a huge shift moment for me.

CHAPTER SUMMARY

In Ayurveda the primordial cause of all disease is forgetting your true nature as spirit, just as Alcoholics Anonymous says that addiction is a spiritual malady. Ayurveda (and Yoga) propose physical remedies and somatic-based care in treating all disease, including addiction, while Western models tend to focus addiction treatment on psychiatric, psychological and increasingly now on pharmacological approaches. Using Ayurvedic principles and practices supports any recovery pathway, empowering individuals in creating and experiencing health and healing as a direct expression of their true light.

SUGGESTED PRACTICE

To introduce an aspect of the lived solution immediately, Yoga of Recovery (YoR) offers an Inner Resource Meditation as our first practice. This comes from iRest (the Integrative Restoration Institute), which is an evidence-based treatment center for pain, addiction and trauma. I suggest you record this short meditation and take up to ten minutes each day to practice it.

Inner Resource: Welcome to the Practice of Inner Resource Meditation[8]

Take time now to develop your *Inner Resource*... this is an Inner Sanctuary that you've visited before, or a brand new place that you're now discovering for the first time... an Inner Sanctuary where you feel totally at ease and secure... able to completely be yourself without concern... This may be a special room... a meadow... a place at the beach... or some other location that when you're here you feel completely protected and secure... or it may simply be the feeling of Being that underlies all that you are... This is your special place or Inner Resource where, when you're here, you can relax and feel completely at ease... allow this imaginative place to arise spontaneously within you as a visual image... accompanied by a felt sense in your body... a feeling of an Inner Sanctuary where you feel secure... protected... at ease... and safe...

Allow all of your senses to come into play... hearing sounds that are soothing and relaxing... perceiving objects that evoke feelings of comfort and ease... perceiving smells and tastes that evoke good feelings... spending time now allowing this inner refuge of comfort, ease and security to blossom completely into your Awareness... experiencing how being here acts on your entire body and mind...

Allow spontaneous associations to arise with your Inner Sanctuary that evoke feelings of security and well-being... objects... animals... people... and other resources that when you perceive them you feel deeply at peace... relaxed... and comfortable... There may be people here who totally support you... value you for who you are... just as you are... Or there may be wisdom figures... a wise man or woman, or a power animal or object... take a few moments now and allow these images to come fully into Awareness along with feelings of comfort, security and ease of being...

Know that you can return to your Inner Resource at a moment's notice... at any time of day or night... you can return whenever you experience the need to feel secure and at ease...

Each day take time to visit your Inner Sanctuary... allow it to become a haven of comfort and ease... so that in your daily life, when you feel distressed by a particular experience... you can pause and visit your Inner Resource and remain here until you feel totally at ease, secure and comfortable... then when you feel ready... return again to the experience and begin meeting, greeting and welcoming it again into Awareness... Knowing that you can return at any time to your inner sanctuary should you desire to feel peaceful and relaxed...

Student Story—New Vocabulary and New Tools

At the recommendation of my Yoga teacher, I committed to the Yoga of Recovery program even though I did not have addictions to substances. Yoga had supported me through some difficult physical and mental challenges. In fact, it was my lifeline during my 30-day hospitalization, allowing me to surrender by centering and focusing on my breath. In the end, YoR was an incredible immersion in self-discovery. Durga used personal experience and stories to motivate us to look at ourselves and our habits through Ayurveda and 12-Step principles. While I wasn't addicted to drinking, nor did I abuse drugs, I was able to see and admit in an honest way that I did have compulsive behaviors and codependency issues that wreaked havoc in my life. In the safe haven of YoR, I became willing to name my dependencies, talk about them and develop a new vocabulary and an authentic and loving inner voice, allowing me to support myself instead of looking for validation from the outside. It can still be a rocky road, but now I have new tools to steer myself back on track when I stray.

Stacy C.

Student Story—Freedom from Pharmaceuticals

Yoga of Recovery helped me break a severe heroin addiction. The exploration of the self—our true nature—through Yoga and Ayurveda guided me through my first 18 months of medication-assisted detox, treatment and recovery. After that first year and a half, I was strong enough and established enough in my recovery to detox off the opioid replacement pharmaceuticals through a month-long Panchakarma treatment in India. Coming off the opioid replacement therapy is not so much of a discussion topic at this time. Allopathic doctors suggest people in recovery from heroin use disorder stay on some form of opioid replacement medicine to avoid a potential relapse. My experience with Yoga and Ayurveda convinced me that the connection I was seeking during my active addiction was not going to come from chemical happiness. The connection I was seeking was within me and the chemicals were only further blocking that connection. After undergoing the deep Panchakarma detoxification, I was free of all pharmaceuticals. As an added bonus I was able to kick the addiction to cigarettes at the same time.

This was in 2015 and I continue with a daily routine built around the Ayurveda diet and lifestyle recommendations, and this has helped me become significantly stronger in my recovery journey. YoR has truly taught me how to "go with the flow." It is a constant practice of contentment and keeping an equanimous state of mind through the ups and downs of daily life—learning to accept and adapt to those ups and downs as they arise has been a big gift for me.

I am now much more patient, tolerant and adaptable to change than I was before. I am now fully comfortable in my own skin in all circumstances and find I can build strength and resilience even in these uncertain times of the world. And any time imbalances arise within me, I know I can turn to the loving care of the suggested practices of YoR.

Shanna D.

ENDNOTES

1   AA (2001) *Alcoholics Anonymous* (4th edn). New York: Alcoholics Anonymous World Services, p. 64; known as the *Big Book of Alcoholics Anonymous*.

2   ibid., p. 24.

3   ibid., p. 45.

4   ibid., p. 64.

5   NIDA (2014) *Drugs, Brains, and Behavior: The Science of Addiction*. www.drugabuse.gov/sites/default/files/soa_2014.pdf

6   NIDA (2020) *The Science of Drug Use and Addiction: The Basics*. www.drugabuse.gov/publications/media-guide/science-drug-use-addiction-basics

7   AA, *Alcoholics Anonymous*, p. 85.

8   The following are original copyrighted works and property of Dr. Richard C. Miller: The iRest Institute Inner Resource. Their use, inclusion and reproduction in this work are granted by license with permission from Dr. Richard C. Miller. Unauthorized reproduction is prohibited. All rights are reserved.

▶ Chapter 2 ◀

AYURVEDA AND RECOVERY

HEALING THE BODY

"I N THE ROOMS," as people in 12-Step programs say, there is a lot of talk about the spiritual solution and the need to find a Higher Power—in truth, what I also needed was something more concrete to guide my day-to-day choices, especially as I was coming up against "new" bad habits and concerns about my behavior once I no longer had alcohol to turn to.

In the early stages of my sobriety, as my pent-up/denied emotions began to thaw out, my tendency was to attempt to change or avoid them with some other distraction. Now that I was aware of the futility of these habits, I had to find a more sustainable way to feel good every day.

What do we do between meetings (of any recovery pathway or sessions with therapists)? And if we practice Yoga, between the mat and the meetings? Ayurveda would provide these answers, and ultimately lead to the creation of a course called YoR: Between the Mat and the Meeting, and this book.

Fully expressed, Ayurveda ("the science of life") is a comprehensive system of medicine, one of the world's oldest and most sophisticated systems of health, practiced and taught by doctors who train for many years. Yet its principles and applications are accessible to everyone and, as such, it is a truly democratic, person-centered life science.

Through self-care, Ayurveda adds the body to our recovery plan, supporting individuals in any circumstances to embody their recovery.

AYURVEDA THREEFOLD CAUSE OF DISEASE

Ayurveda texts explain that from the spiritual root of all disease (forgetting our true nature is spirit) stems a threefold cause of disease:

1. misuse of the senses.

2. failure of the intellect/crimes against wisdom.

3. the effects of time/environment.

These three seemingly simple concepts are actually quite extraordinary. In addition to making sense on their own, I immediately recognized how they correlated with AA's Big Book on this topic of the causes of alcoholism (that can be extended to cover all addictions). What I found was that these two paths shared similar perspectives on the disease of addiction. The Big Book describes these three components of alcoholism, which distinguish it from situational or occasional heavy drinking—that it is:

▸ an allergy of the body

▸ an obsession of the mind[1]

▸ a progressive (and fatal) illness.[2]

This changed everything for me. While they used different phrasing, the foundational ideas in each system—Ayurveda and AA/12-Step programs—aligned and I could see how they applied to my own experience with addiction and recovery.

1. Misuse of the Senses: An Allergy and Phenomenon of Craving

The allergy concept was the key that opened the door for me to understand and accept my issue with alcohol. The *Big Book of Alcoholics Anonymous* describes the problem of alcoholism as a "manifestation of an allergy" from which arises a "phenomenon of craving"[3] that becomes "paramount to all other interests."[4] Hence, we become "seriously ill, bodily and mentally."[5]

The solution AA proposes is complete abstinence from alcohol (or drug of choice/trigger food/behavior in other 12-Step programs). This is because the reported experience of many who suffer is that they have "one symptom in common: they cannot start drinking without developing the phenomenon of craving."[6]

This described the way I experienced my problem with alcohol: once I start, I can't stop. I didn't drink every day, I never drank in the morning—the hair of the dog didn't work for me; often I was too sick to keep anything down. It was a truth I recognized at once—my issue was the first drink, pure and simple—so astoundingly simple! All I had to do was not take that first drink and I'd never again have to deal with all the issues and consequences that came from my drunken behavior.

I can recall the feeling that activated when alcohol entered my system and I felt its initial effects. AA says the allergy manifests as a phenomenon of craving and that is exactly what I experienced. It felt like a switch was flipped, a light going on—game on! But I had no control over how much I would drink and consequently I'd often do or say things that caused a lot of guilt, remorse and shame.

Other people could have fun and know when to stop, why couldn't I? I accepted this allergy perspective as it related so closely to my experience. It was simple enough to grasp and build the needed change around. It was not rocket science: just don't take the first drink.

2. Failure of the Intellect/Crimes against Wisdom: Control, Obsession, Insanity

I just wanted to be like everyone else, go out, kick up my heels, have a good time, have a good laugh but... there was a drag, a darkness in this for me. I was in emotional pain around certain aspects of my life and alcohol seemed to provide a release from that worry, tension and fear. It allowed me to be free, uninhibited, more bold and confident, but there was a high price to pay for the good effects that were so temporary while the ill effects were becoming a more stable feature of my life.

When deep in the pain of hangovers (which would leave me throwing up for up to eight hours the next day), I would desperately try to picture a new me where this no longer happened, but it was simply not within my sights. There were always some obstacles obscuring the possibility of that becoming a reality. The alcohol acted like a strong central nervous system depressant. I was in the pits regularly, full of self-loathing, baffled as to how I was becoming the thing I most hated.

Consider this quote from the Big Book: "The idea that somehow, someday he will control and enjoy his drinking is the great obsession of every abnormal drinker. The persistence of this illusion is astonishing. Many pursue it into the gates of insanity or death."[7]

You can replace the word "drinking" with your addiction/recovery focus; the faulty thought processes operate in the same way. It is clear here that the disease of addiction includes both a physical component and a psychological one. We literally know better yet act contrary to this knowing.

THE MIND AND CONTROL

In order to stay in control, I, like most people with substance use disorder, had come up with strategies and made bargains with myself, creating and then breaking "rules" around what was acceptable or allowable. 12-Step programs take the perspective that reducing or curtailing does not work, because we'll always break our agreements; hence, 12-Step programs state that "the only relief we have to suggest is entire abstinence."[8]

Of course, this has always been surrounded by debate in many areas of our society and there are several points that are worth considering. I recommend you read web articles from the late Dr. Alan Marlatt, the founder of Harm Reduction, where he discusses the limitations of abstinence-only interventions especially given the stigma, and criminal justice implications addicts face when seeking help. He says, "We'll help you, whatever your goal is. You want to quit, we'll help you. You want to cut back, we'll help you. We're not going to shut you out" (www.psychotherapy.net/interview/marlatt-harm-reduction). Also, there are newer organizations like the Chicago Recovery Alliance (CRA), a racially and ethnically diverse group who provide a wide array of options for achieving "any positive change" for those living with HIV and drug use and reducing drug related harm, especially overdose deaths (https://anypositivechange.org).

These are very important considerations when looking at state and medical interventions. However, 12-Step programs were always meant to be for the individual to choose; they were not intended to be medically, court or state mandated. They are mutual help organizations based on peer support with no professional therapy. This is one of their unique contributions—they are free and available 24/7 worldwide.

My attempts to control my addiction through limiting required so much mental effort and it never worked. Once I became sober, I used a lot of the same "control" strategies around other substances and behaviors, including a love for sugar, but it was always distressing at how quickly I had to renegotiate my own best intended boundaries with myself.

However, my efforts to create control were also on a positive track. I did have an aspiration to feel good and rid myself of this crazy behavior. I took up Yoga, watched my diet and read self-help books. I could connect with a healthier, more loving part of myself briefly but never consistently for any length of time. I was always just a first drink away from more demoralizing self-sabotage.

THE WISDOM TO KNOW THE DIFFERENCE

In my own recovery, I found this concept of "crimes against wisdom" to be very freeing and empowering. I woke up to the notion that this behavior did not come from outside myself. The "crime" was against my own wisdom, my own consciousness—my own sense of self, right and wrong, my own inner compass.

While I might be finding ways to rationalize my behavior away, the real, deeper truth was that it was just not okay with me—these non-life-promoting behaviors went against my own inner intention for my life. Addiction dimmed/obscured my inner light.

This well-known Serenity Prayer serves as a focal point for 12-Step group members: "God, grant me the serenity to accept the things I cannot change, courage to change the things I can, and wisdom to know the difference." This "crimes against wisdom" idea indicated to me that the "wisdom to know the difference" was within me.

I didn't need someone to tell me how to think and behave, that knowledge was within me, for my own sense of purpose and thriving. I did not need to be converted or instructed in someone else's way, but to find a way to connect with the wisdom within me.

Ayurveda supports this inner wisdom within each of us, the inner light that shines steadily and guides us forward. We'll look more at how in Chapter 3, which goes into more detail on the concept of the gunas.

3. Effects of Time: Progressive Illness

PROGRESSIVE AND FATAL

I first experienced the pitiful and incomprehensible demoralization aspect of alcoholism in my mother as I watched her slow suicide from drinking over 20 years. It was awful to hear her crying and repeating "I wish I were dead" when she was under the influence.

As my own drinking and out-of-balance lifestyle progressed into my early, mid, then late 20s, my lows got ever more desperate and despairing and the laughs and enjoyable highs got less and less frequent and lasted for a shorter time. I also lost externals—jobs and boyfriends. I could see and feel the downward spiral, and the further down I went the more hopeless I felt that I'd ever be able to pull myself out of it. It would be easier to succumb to my fate, I thought, and a large part of me wanted to, at certain times, when I was unable to see any other way out. I recognize myself in this statement from the AA Big Book, and felt the heartbreaking reality of it in the story of my mother's illness: "All of us felt at times that we were regaining control, but such intervals—usually brief—were inevitably followed by still less control, which led in time to pitiful and incomprehensible demoralization. We are convinced... that alcoholics of our type are in the grip of a progressive illness. Over any considerable period we get worse, never better."[9]

Yet at other times, I forged ahead, making new attempts at claiming a happy, successful life. That all ended when my mother died suddenly from a heart attack. She had reached the fatal part—it was shocking and so final. This was the disaster I had been trying to avert since I first foresaw it at 12 years old. Now at 32 years old it was a grim reality. She was gone, and all chance of her reclaiming her health and happiness, all chance of us having a close mother-daughter relationship, were gone. It was a blow that left me reeling.

My alcoholism gained strength. I was bereft and so lost, I became ever more reckless and aggressive-depressive. I really couldn't care less anymore. My mother died in July 1997 and I was finally fired from my job in December 1997. My actions and behaviors meant I could barely show up for anything after that. I could not pull it together in any coherent way; the fabric of my life was fraying away and I could not stop it. My nature under the influence ranged from vicious to pathetically maudlin.

I moved to the USA in March 1998 and continued in a downward spiral. I went to my first meeting of AA in the USA nine months after I arrived, in December 1998. My last drink of alcohol was New Year's Eve 1998. My clean and sober sobriety date is 22 November 1999. It took 17 months after my mother died for me to fully and consistently choose sobriety. I came to see that my story of alcoholism was often inseparable from my mother's—that was my inner truth. Her death released both her and me. She went to her grave and I went into a free-fall dive to my bottom, which led me to sobriety through AA, a return to a Hatha Yoga practice, and eventually to Ayurveda. In the end, her death saved my life.

ONE DAY AT A TIME

There is a great time sickness in our world. In the West particularly, we plan a lot of our time, we worry about it, don't seem to have enough of it; we kill time, save time and, of course, monetize it, measuring our worth by how much money we can trade an hour of our time for. Time is linear, marching ever forward as the past gets dusty. We also have enormous denial around time, living as though we will go on forever, conveniently setting aside the notion that our unique span of time will come to an end.

One of the brilliant aspects of Ayurveda medicine is that we can begin to see the movement of time as an ally. Ayurveda shines a light on the cyclical nature of time and supports more natural energy expenditure through the timing of essential daily tasks and habits. Through Ayurveda, we use time to create a pattern of self-care working with the qualities of our stage of life, where we are in recovery, the season of the year, etc.

A primary message of AA is to take it—life and recovery—one day at a time. As we saw above, Ayurveda recognizes that the effects of time and environment are a significant factor in the manifestation as well as the aggravation and progression of a disease. We will return to this potent concept through Ayurveda many times in these pages.

AYURVEDA PRACTICES CONTRIBUTE TO SUSTAINED RECOVERY

How do we bring Ayurveda into our daily lives in layered ways that we can tailor to our circumstances and innate tendencies? How do we embody a lived solution?

The three causes of disease each point to their own solutions. At the end of many of the chapters ahead, you will find suggested Ayurveda practices, small routines to try out and experience, all of which counter each of these causes of disease. Together, they support the natural health and harmony of our mind-body systems and provide a welcome, and often much-needed, complement to any recovery pathway in addressing our day-to-day embodied experiences.

1. Sense-able recovery. Through Ayurveda we make use of daily, body-based self-care routines to address "misuse of the senses" and bring our organic systems into balance. In Chapter 6, we will look more closely at how we act out using our senses—and how we can start to establish more awareness and balance through Ayurveda.

2. The gunas and the nature of the mind. Ayurveda provides keen insight into how the mind works and how we can use that knowledge to prevent—or undo—all those crimes against wisdom! Further along in this book, we will see how practices like meditation and consistent routine help to slow our automatic reactions and steady our sense of self.

3. Natural rhythms and flow. Ayurveda makes a connection between our biologies and the patterns and rhythms of nature, inside and around us, bringing awareness to the "effects of time and environment." Primarily by working with the qualities of the elements, we can mitigate negative effects and promote a state of flow instead. For many in recovery, this has provided a true breakthrough and we will investigate this further in Chapter 12.

CHAPTER SUMMARY

Many approaches to recovery in the West tend to overlook the physical body. Ayurveda identifies three causes of disease and treats and cares for the body as a foundation for healing, suggesting healthy new self-care routines and habits for body and mind as well as a holistic model for understanding ourselves within time and space. It offers an embodied **design for living** that supports recovery and empowers us in creating health and well-being in all aspects of our lives.

SUGGESTED PRACTICE

Time sickness is the ultimate lifestyle disorder. Do you relate to time in a dysfunctional way? Do you feel like there is never enough time in the day, that you're racing against time? Do you fear aging? It's not about time but the mismatch between your perception and reality. Journal about this now for about 15 minutes. I also recommend the Chopra 21-Day Meditation Series "Making Every Moment Matter."[10]

Student Story—Healing My Heart

After beating lymphatic cancer in 2020, I decided to take greater responsibility for my overall health by choosing the path of sobriety. I grew up in an addictive home with divorced parents and I started abusing substances at 16 years old, my top choice being alcohol. These quick fixes would sedate me until I was sober again and the sorrow that I was wrestling with the day before returned. For years my depression worsened and I found myself repeating the same self-destructive patterns. Though I was able to recognize that I was living in a loop I did not know what to do to change the course of my life. It felt like insanity masked by a smile.

Eventually, the drinking began to cause physical discomfort, particularly in the lymph nodes around my neck. I saw a doctor about the pain and a biopsy confirmed that I had stage 2b Nodular Sclerosis Hodgkin's Lymphoma at 25 years old. The doctors couldn't find the cause of my cancer, making me believe the issue went deeper than what could be understood by modern Western medicine. Scans revealed that my cancer was encroaching on my heart and I took this as a message from my body that this is where my healing needed to begin, in my heart.

I remained sober during my treatments, but after, it did not take long for all of the old issues with substances and people to return. I was still in denial about the cause of my drinking and escapist tactics. I quickly decided to put an end to the madness. I had seen alcohol ruin enough lives and I was not about to let it take me too, not after the year of chemotherapy treatments I had endured. I gave up drinking for the New Year and very quickly saw my life begin to shift. It made me wonder what life could be like if I fully decided to stay sober and really deal with the heartache that had been following me since I was a little girl.

Three months into my sobriety, I was blessed to find the Yoga of Recovery program. It offered the guidance and support that I needed to live a more clear and intentional life, especially in the early phases of sobriety. I found empathetic support in the YoR community, people who understood me and served as hopeful lights for what was waiting for me down the road. The Ayurvedic tools empowered me to make decisions that serve my highest good long term. YoR helped me understand the root cause of my afflictions and addictions, and showed me how to take loving action to improve the quality of my life experience. In the end, my experience with cancer made me stronger and helped me believe that there was a healthier way to work with myself and my emotions. I am now freer in thought and action than ever before and happy to finally and fully be sober.

Darienne M.

Student Story – With Ayurveda It Feels Like I've Come Home

I experienced my nature as extreme, both in addiction and recovery. My driving internal message was "more, more, more". I had tried almost everything and was interested in Eastern philosophy (Yoga and mindfulness) even during my addicted behaviors; then I came across Ayurveda. It calmed me and it was simple. Yoga and meditation help me find the inner consciousness and deepen my connection with my higher power.

At eight years sober I felt that myself and others (both recovering people and the general population) were somewhat "manic" when it came to self-care regimens, whether it be running, going to the gym or becoming obsessed and strict with the latest fad diet. With so many people modeling "extreme" behavior around me, I was easily influenced to feel that this was the way to tackle my new life in recovery too. However, this only brought me to exhaustion.

Ayurveda tells me not to be extreme – to seek "the middle way". I can relax and trust myself, obey the odd food craving and not hold myself to such enforced and rigid diet and exercise routines. If I really want some chocolate or pizza then I just have it, in moderation. Better that than to obsess about it for the next few hours. I feel it harps back to traditional ways – our old style of living where you've got your food and herbal medicines and what you do when you get up in the morning – you do it and you leave it there, and go about your day without obsessing over every detail. It's been an amazing circular thing for me, it's taken me back to the comfort of home-cooked food – things that used to pacify me as a child. With Ayurveda it feels like I've come home. I keep it simple: my attitude to life, my spirituality, my general health. I have a routine. I get up and pray and make my bed, oil my skin, meditate and then shower, etc. Ayurveda offers me a natural way of living, a comfortable routine. It's brilliant because it is moderate which is the best mantra for a person in recovery – "moderate not manic". Now I can more easily see when I am moving toward old behaviors and doing things to the extreme, and I can also see it in others and choose my company and advice from people who live a more moderate life!

Rachael B

ENDNOTES

1   AA, *Alcoholics Anonymous*, p. 355.
2   ibid., p. 30.
3   ibid., p. xxiv.
4   ibid., p. xxv.
5   ibid., p. 7.
6   ibid., p. xxvi.
7   ibid., p. 30.
8   ibid.
9   ibid.
10 https://chopracentermeditation.com

▶ Chapter 3 ◀

THE GUNAS

IT WAS DURING MY SECOND VISIT TO THE ASHRAM—18 months sober and in a 12-Step program—that I heard the phrase "crimes against wisdom," and it had a huge impact on me. One of its main appeals was that the phrase is not "sins against God" as the God topic is constantly and hotly debated in 12-Step programs. Ayurveda is a non-theistic philosophy. Its view of the body-mind helped me understand that wisdom is within each one of us (Sanskrit term is buddhi), as we are all connected to Universal Intelligence (Sanskrit term is mahat).

The history of addiction treatment in the West has been marred by the belief that addicts are bad people who need to become good. There have been decades of effort to change this to the idea of addicts being sick people who need to get well. I have always appreciated the deeper psychology of both Ayurveda and Yoga which can add the view of the addict as a seeker who is ultimately looking for the supreme joy of our true, essential nature or self-realization, albeit by inappropriate means.

Our true, essential nature stems from universal life force/intelligence and from that everything operates under the law of karma (all actions incur an equal and corresponding reaction). Remembrance of our true nature as spirit helps us stay balanced while operating, active and fully alive, in the world.

David Frawley's books, *Ayurveda and the Mind* and *Yoga and Ayurveda*, guide what we'll be looking at around Ayurvedic psychology—I highly recommend you read these books and all other books by David Frawley.

According to Ayurveda, the main cause of division and disease is the ego— our sense of separation. Of course, this again relates to the primordial cause of disease being our forgetfulness of our true nature as spirit. Ayurveda views our mind through connected component parts: consciousness as the source of our life force (prana), which gives rise to the buddhi (which is translated into English as "intellect") and ego (the "I" process—the sense of separation) through which we engage with our world through our mind and senses.

Each of us has our own portion of Universal Intelligence operating within us. For our purposes, rather than refer to buddhi by its usual English translation of intellect, let's refer to it as "wise mind" as it represents our individual portion of Universal Intelligence (mahat). Ideally this "wise mind" guides the ego and sense mind, which tend to draw us out into the external world. This is certainly encouraged at every opportunity in our modern consumerist culture and most of us feel the ill effects of this in our habits of comparing and despairing, competing and craving. The sense mind externalizes our sense of self and we measure ourselves according to material things. When the wise mind is guiding us we are able to be more discerning and live a life of dignity, making choices that support who we truly are at a deeper level of self-awareness.

THE PSYCHOLOGY OF AYURVEDA

In understanding the mind, Ayurveda uses the model of the three gunas. Here are some of the definitions of the gunas I relate to (from David Frawley's books[1]):

▸ The gunas are the primal forces/qualities of nature which are the main powers of Universal Intelligence.

▸ All objects in the universe consist of various combinations of the gunas. They are the most subtle qualities of nature that underlie matter, life and mind.

▸ Ayurveda uses the gunas to determine mental and spiritual nature.

The three gunas are the causal energies of creation behind the mind, and ideas of balance, motion and resistance. They are the energies through which our mind and deeper consciousness function.

We will be looking at the gunas in depth in this and future chapters, but in brief: the three gunas are Sattva, Rajas and Tamas:

▸ Sattva is the quality of intelligence.

▸ Rajas is the quality of energy/activity.

▸ Tamas is the quality of materiality.

Relieve Me of the Bondage of Self

In the 12-Step program, participants often speak of their ego problems. The ACA program (Adult Children of Alcoholic and Dysfunctional families) specifically states that our

> families [world, culture, community] were not safe enough for us to feel comfortable in being ourselves. Thus, we isolate ourselves by burying, hiding, denying, abandoning, and betraying our True Self and presenting a false self to the world. From this protective space we could keep our fear of people at an acceptable level. We didn't allow many folks the opportunity to hurt us, and when they were able to get close, any separation produced an almost intolerable feeling of pain that led us to refortify our defenses and to further isolate ourselves from any intimacy.[2]

I believe that this provides a very succinct perspective on the fundamental struggle at the bottom of all problems around addictiveness: it occurs at the level of our own self-identity, our roles and our essential safety in relation to others.

The word gunas means "what binds." Ayurveda doctor and author Robert Svoboda offers an understanding of self-identity/ego from the perspective of the three gunas that I have found particularly useful:[3]

▸ Sattva is the internalizing "I," our more conscious sense of interconnected self.

▸ Rajas is the externalizing "I," the active "I," always on the move, searching for something with which to self-identify.

▸ Tamas is the objectifying "I," our least conscious sense of self, often overly identified with the body.

Our Faulty Perceptual Process

Our forgetting of our true nature causes us to digress into faulty perceptual processes which contribute to all the imbalances we experience in our mind-body system. We have made use of the gunas questionnaire (see the back of this book) to help us gauge our current perceptual process.

UNDERSTANDING THE GUNAS: THE MIND AS A LAKE

Here is a helpful analogy for understanding the influence of each of the gunas on our minds. I find this lake analogy of the mind helps me to picture the different capacities of the mind under the influence of the different Gunic qualities.

A Sattvic Mind

In Sattva, we have a still, clear lake. Its surface is like a mirror that reflects the things around it. It gives a very clear picture because the surface is calm, so the reflection is stable and reliable. A Sattvic mind has clarity; the light of consciousness shines through clearly and steadily. A Sattvic mind can observe the emotions but detach from them. This is what we attempt to do when we sit to meditate: we will notice the thoughts and the emotions that come up, we observe and let them pass. The thoughts are still there but we don't dwell on them or cling to them.

A Rajasic Mind

Now take this same lake and let's look at it in its Rajasic nature when the activity of the thoughts creates a disturbance, like waves on the surface. The objects surrounding the lake are still the same, but now we see a distorted picture because of the movement on the surface of the lake. The waves represent the emotions and thought waves. It is the same lake, the same scenery, but the activity on the surface of the lake has changed. In Rajas, we tend to identify with the emotions. We get caught up in the drama of life and our emotions tend to be expressed reactively without much thought.

A Tamasic Mind

Some of these waves have been big enough to disturb the sediment at the bottom of the lake, which results in dark, murky water. This is Tamas. Again, the actual scenery remains the same, but there is very little reflection because of the darkness on the surface. In Tamas, the emotions tend to be suppressed and repressed. Most of us have some aspects where we have this murkiness, areas where we haven't quite done the house cleaning; it's a little dark and shadowy in that part of our life, so we steer clear of it. It may be that we are secretive, hiding parts of ourselves, cut off from the sunlight of the spirit.

It is important to see that this is the same lake under different conditions. The mind has the capacity, in its Sattvic nature, to become clear, calm, steady, harmonious with its environment, because it is reflecting the inner light. It also has the capacity to become Rajasic: with so many thoughts and emotions, confusion reigns and we become reactive, attacking and defending to protect our point of view. Then Tamas comes with its heavy and dark qualities. Now we are refusing to deal with things, moving into denial and resistance.

Here is another quick and helpful interpretation of the meaning of each guna:

- ▶ Sattva—revealing.

- ▶ Rajas—projecting.

- ▶ Tamas—veiling.

THE MIND AND ADDICTION

As the gunas are formative to our whole consciousness we'll base our reframing of our story of addiction and its solution around them. Dr. Svoboda speaks about how it is the nature of humans to create narrative; healers listen deeply then help to reweave the story.

Reframing Our "Addictiveness" Narratives

We tend to live through our senses, which have an outgoing nature. This is the nature of Rajas; its movement is outward. Our society encourages hyper-speed and hyper-stimulation of the senses. Everywhere we go, there is advertising, and reminders of things that we could be eating or buying or doing. In our modern consumerist culture we are at the mercy of a powerful advertising industry with very tempting ways to entice us. The sense pleasures are amplified—and constantly shouting—trying to grab our attention. Yoga says we can consider the senses like five powerful horses: they tend to run wild and can rule our lives. We are at their mercy. The more we live a life based on ego, the more we will be following our sensual desires.

In our regular daily lives, we expend our energy in work, travel, exercise, play and entertainment (TV, computers, movies, games, podcasts, social media etc.). We receive a lot of information through the senses, yet we only have so much energy so at some point we may begin to feel tired. This is a "symptom" that comes up: "I'm tired." What happens then? If you take some rest in response to that message then this would be the Sattvic choice. No drama, no resistance, we simply observe the feeling and know how to remedy it: for the feeling of tiredness, a short rest is appropriate.

> In Yoga of Recovery, we make use of body sensing and breath sensing to help us simply be with and accept the sensations that arise throughout the day in a more Sattvic way. You'll find a simple breath awareness practice at the end of this chapter. I wish to acknowledge that the general outline of these come from my training in iRest.org

However, what we tend to do instead is reach for stimulation, something that pushes the system back into action. We all do it to some extent, and this is often because our action is based in self-seeking, self-will—maybe even "self-will run riot"[4] (as it says in the AA Big Book), even in recovery. We act from a "what's in it for me" outlook—just as the marketers model to us: how much can we make or take (money, power, prestige, possessions). We are driven by our ambitions, desires and fears and this causes us to increasingly move into a state of fragmentation (Rajasic ego). Our lives are ruled by ego, described by David Frawley as the "I" fabrication process. Even if the mind does come up with the idea of taking a break or a simple walk to help our energy, we often ignore our own good idea as we are so driven and externalized in this world.

Remember the second cause of disease—"crimes against wisdom." The injunction on these "crimes" does not come from outside ourselves. The crime is against our own wisdom, our own consciousness and wise mind, our inherent sense of self, right and wrong, our own inner compass. While we can find ways to rationalize away our behavior, we cannot actually hide from the truth that is not okay with us. Our choice to ignore our truth goes against our own inner light and guidance, which want us to thrive.

We ignore the quieter wise mind that counters the loud demands of the ego and sense mind. We ignore our own inwardly generated sound advice. We listen to this voice that provides a reason why we should resort again to improper action. This is the cunning, baffling and powerful nature of the addiction process: we hear the whispers of our own inner wisdom, yet we decide to ignore it. Dr. Robert Svoboda summarizes this scenario with the following statement: "Inaccurate perceptions encourage tighter bondage; proper perception promotes freedom."[5]

Mostly the mind behaves like a highly expensive lawyer, but it is arguing with itself. Our wise mind knows we are tired and would benefit from rest, but then the "lawyer mind" kicks in and says if we rest then this might happen or that may not happen so we cannot rest, because the universe depends on us! We have to show up, there are things that we must get, there are things we can't afford to lose and we worry about what other people think of us. We all have this tendency of the mind: the next time it happens, tune in and listen and notice that it's often using the past and the future for its case. It offers reasons from the past (distant or recent) of why we deserve this, and/ or it will convince us to make the wise choice tomorrow. The "lawyer mind" persuades us to just go ahead with this unwise choice today.

The result is that we experience more and more imbalanced symptoms of the Rajasic mind such as fear, worry, anxiety, anger, irritation, judgment, blame, greed, attachment. The more we ignore our inner wisdom, the more we experience this as an almost constant mental/emotional state. At this stage, often what happens is that the substances and behaviors we initially used for stimulation are no longer enough. As Dr. Gabor Maté says: "It is hard to get enough of something that almost works." We start to need things with stronger effects. And why? Just because we have ignored our own inner wisdom.

When we employ rationalization and justification, the double trouble is that we are paying this expensive lawyer with our own life force energy (prana). Initially it does take quite a bit of mental energy to argue against the care of the system, allowing the self-destructive choice to win today's case. However, as long as it is allowed to happen and the more it happens, then the likelihood is that the mind starts to drop down into Tamas, the lower level of consciousness that sustains and turns a blind eye to this corrupted activity. In Tamas, these behaviors become more ingrained and habitual; they proceed without much pre-thought, so they become harder to recognize or change. There is dullness, apathy, inertia. We're at the stage now where the expensive lawyer inside the head doesn't even need to argue the case; we just succumb to the idea that this is the only option open to us. We've actually spent so much of our energy on this rationalization and justification that we have little left for new ideas or change.

Here we are reaching the state of addiction, and with the addiction comes denial, desperation, despair, delusion, depression, disintegration, decay and possibly, ultimately, death. Over the long term, we may need to use stronger drugs or more regularly as we feel almost devoid of vitality. We go from self-seeking action to lethargy and heaviness. Our life is an emotional rollercoaster. We constantly need something to stimulate us into action so we can perform in a Rajasic mode for a while before we fall back down into Tamas. A whole cocktail and combination of substances, behaviors and distractions may be employed at different times of the day to manage this precarious system. Deepak Chopra describes addiction in these five words: "when more is never enough."

THE OUT AND DOWN OF ADDICTION

The movement of Tamas is downward. It is interesting that the phrase "the down and out of addiction" has been coined; actually the journey is more "out and down." We act out so many times with more and more substances and behaviors involved. We've gone out, out, out—right to the edge—and then something tips us over the edge.

This is the baffling part, because no one really knows what that something is going to be. We may have the idea that we're holding it all together, feeling okay, and then something happens. It is often remarked that it is not life's major dramas, but some small thing that becomes the "straw that broke the camel's back."

Our actions have been creating an ongoing, cumulative effect on a weakening system that is becoming more and more susceptible to stress but we've been ignoring or disguising the distress symptoms with anything we can get our hands on. The trouble is that while the things we resort to actually do give some amount of stimulation or pleasure, it is only for the short term. In the long term these escapes result in deeper disturbances that sustain craving and insatiable desire, hence we rarely reach the point where the feel-good effects outweigh the suffering caused by these choices. We are increasingly in persistent pain, suffering, distress and conflict, yet we keep doing the same thing—reaching for the short-term pleasure, even while being fairly certain of the long-term pain that results from our actions. This is defined in 12 Steps as insanity (or worded more gently, as lack of clarity): doing the same thing over and over and expecting different results. This is Tamas. This mind resists the light; it's gone into hiding and it's secretive as denial is our way of protecting ourselves from a change we feel is impossible. We are often mired in guilt and shame, secrets and lies. Our mind's ability to self-regulate at this level is very low.

A Moment of Clarity

Yet somehow in all this darkness, there is a moment of clarity. Actually, it's likely there have been many moments of clarity that have been ignored but this time the message gets through: "I really shouldn't do this, I can't do this again, no more, I can't continue like this."

It is reported by many that this is the turning point; somehow we realize that our situation is quite dire and we become willing, often reluctantly, to try something different, to change direction. When that happens, many people head into the 12 Steps or into therapy with a counselor or Yoga therapist.

From I to We

The good news is that "we" is the antidote to the "I" of the ego and isolation. "We" is also the first word of the 12 Steps. As soon as we show up, to a meeting or a session, we are working with that little chink of light that's coming through—and Sattva is that light. It represents our connection with the wisdom within us, the Universal Intelligence. Remember darkness is not an absence of light; it is the veiling of the light. We all have the light within us. We can reclaim our connection to wisdom. How do we do that? The best medicine for crimes against wisdom is the company of the wise. In Yoga, this is called satsang: to be in the company of the wise/wisdom holders, with the truth seekers.

One of the first recommendations of action given to new members by 12-Step programs is to attend meetings regularly (90 meetings in 90 days) and to commit to service. These suggestions counter our habitual pattern of selfish, self-seeking action and can almost immediately lift us up out of the swamp of our own self-created misery.

Initially, in the early stages when Tamas dominates, it is likely that we will need a lot of supervision. Left to our own devices, it is too easy to opt out into our exiled state of desperate aloneness and terminal uniqueness. Just showing up helps alleviate the hold the Tamas has. We show up among people who are living the solution to a problem that has us floored, people who have been through similar scrapes and struggles. We hear them share their stories and we can identify, and through that we become willing and teachable.

FROM PATHOLOGY TO POTENTIAL

It is important to continuously remind ourselves of the hopeful message of empowerment that a holistic health system like Ayurveda offers, especially in a society dominated by a disease-based medical model. The mind, like the lake under the different conditions, has the capacity, in its Sattvic nature, to reflect the inner light of consciousness. The waves and murky conditions play out on that lake. The soul is always there. Clarity, calm and consciousness exist and with some concerted and supervised efforts, we can find a way to calm the storm of our emotions and connect more clearly with wisdom.

The gunas illustrate our reason for hope for healing, outlined beautifully by David Frawley in one of his lectures in this description:

- Sattva—self-mastery.

- Rajas—active development.

- Tamas—latent potential.

Ayurveda offers us a dynamic picture of both balance and imbalance. In my opinion, we should question any labels we are given—they may be helpful for an immediate need but watch out that we don't live up to our labels. The message of Ayurveda is Potential, not just Pathology.

MY PERSONAL STORY: THE VELOCITY OF ESCAPE

In his book *Between the World and Me*, Ta-Nehisi Coates describes how television showed him images of "other worlds" and how he knew that his:

> portion of the American galaxy, where bodies were enslaved by a tenacious gravity, was black and that the other, liberated portion was not. I knew that some inscrutable energy preserved the breach. I felt, but did not yet understand, the relation between that other world and me. And I felt in this a cosmic injustice, a profound cruelty, which infused an abiding, irrepressible desire to unshackle my body and achieve the velocity of escape.[6]

Although we grew up in different continents, and there are many very apparent differences between his life circumstances and mine, his phrase "the velocity of escape" deeply resonates with me—it's a perfect summary of a realization I had years ago regarding my life and the gunas. Growing up, my household had been affected by grief and loss in many ways. Both my parents were from Scotland and had met and married in New Jersey, USA. My father died at 44 years old, leaving my mother with five children aged between three and nine years old. She resolutely moved us all back to Scotland within two months of his death. Initially we lived with her parents, but her own mother reproached her life choices with disapproval summed up in the statement, "you made your bed, now lie in it." We moved to a tenement apartment close by and my mum worked full time in a factory while we all went to school. Her relationship with her mother continued to be marred by this unsympathetic and harsh judgment. As life presented my mother with numerous challenges—trying to make ends meet, ensuring our education and taking care of us through numerous health challenges, she became increasingly unavailable to us as she was so tired, worn out and fearful.

The television showed us class and labor battles alongside fantasy life, which for me were the TV shows "Little House on the Prairie" and "The Waltons." I feel these shows warped my sense of reality, because they showed me an illusion that I believed to be true: troubles came but everyone pulled together and the issues were all summarily resolved, agreeably and lovingly. In my life, I prayed and prayed and nothing ever seemed to resolve; the problems kept coming and it felt like they would last forever. My mother became even more unavailable as she drank more and more. By the age of 11, I had formed a strong codependent mission around her. I became aware that she had a drinking problem and I was obsessed with controlling it or battling against it, and she reacted to my hypervigilance and scathing judgment with both verbal and physical abuse. Despair felt like a never-ending cycle, whereas joy was so fleeting and fast, so transient. I recognized the "tenacious gravity" Ta-Nehisi refers to. I have a strong memory of scenes in TV shows that had a person sinking into quicksand. I think my subconscious perception of life had that feeling: the enormous effort that was needed to not get pulled under.

In my early teens I understood that I needed to achieve the "velocity of escape" from the effects of alcoholism in my home life. However, the more my home life became disrupted, the less confident and courageous I felt to break away from it, while at the same time feeling all the more desperate to be free of it. I needed to get out to survive. My first suicide attempt was around 14 years old; it was an extreme response but I arrived at that kind of thinking quite young. Deep down I knew I could not win against the irrational decisions and interpersonal conflicts of the people around me and no one listened to a word I had to say.

I did everything I could to get approval and feel safe but I got neither. I was ridiculed for trying to belong elsewhere, with people outside of the family. "Blood is thicker than water," they would say. Outside my home, my friends, their parents and my teachers liked me and seemed to enjoy my company. I felt part of things and positive around them but my mother/family continuously told me that they'd drop me, that they could not be trusted. I was to stick to my own type and not "rise above my station." I had a strong need to belong and I loved my family, but I was innately unable to settle for what seemed to me to be unreasonable constrictions.

These conditions set up for me a need for alcohol as the rocket fuel through which I could get out—achieve the "velocity of escape." The Rajas effect of what alcohol could do attracted me as it offered me a ticket out of the feeling of futility and heaviness of my home life. I also enjoyed the Tamas effect of alcohol—it let me forget and numb out the emotional pain I felt around my conflicted emotions. Mostly I craved it for its power to give me the courage to express myself more boldly and to seek and walk through a door to freedom and opportunity. I hardened myself and fired up my resolve to get out and never re-create the downtrodden resignation and despair around me. I can now recognize this despair as a factor of the intergenerational trauma caused by the adverse community experiences and addictions that had affected my parents and grandparents—the grief and hardships of loss of family members, rationing and evacuation of children that occurred during World War II, alco-holism and the financial stress of being working class within the entrenched class system of Great Britain.

I had been told that I needed to be nice; it was important to be liked. I should study to pass exams, get qualified so I could get a good job, find a good partner and then I'd be happy. I went about achieving these things but to my dismay, I could not say I was happy. The heartache of the progressive reper-cussions of alcoholism in my family and myself was like a fog that just would not lift. It felt like I was shackled to misery. It looked like I had flown the nest but emotionally I was unable to shake the feeling of rejection and fear that haunted me from my family of origin issues, even though I had "escaped" to London and was now hundreds of miles away from them. Nothing quenched my thirst for wanting to feel whole.

This sense of abandonment was my "hole in the soul" that nothing could fill. It is my primal wound. In some sense, the "God" thing made it worse. Believing and trusting in a God that allowed these things to happen seemed ridiculous. As a child I had done what the priests and religious people told me to do: I prayed—and things got worse. To me, it was obvious that I had to renounce prayer, faith and belief and make my own way. Of course, this left me fighting and struggling in the "real world," overly dependent on externals for support: money, friends, the people who had the power and prestige etc.

Every time I reached a new level of achievement, I was disappointed at how hollow it felt. Now I recognize that this was because I was trying to resolve my soul hunger with external material success. However, if I dared mention that to anyone, I was just encouraged to work toward the next goal. The idea that a carrot could be dangled and I'd trot along behind also became increasingly ridiculous. I could not shake the memory of the emptiness of previous goals I'd reached, so the carrot didn't work so well.

I knew I needed my job so I could be independent; it was crucially impor-tant for me to not need anyone. I wanted a partner so I could be loved, but I was unable to love myself; my alcoholism made me hate myself, so I could not receive love from another and trust it. Everything I was seeking in life was meant to provide me with a sense of security, but nothing did. I can now see that is because it all came from fear, survival of the separate self (ego), and the solutions were all externals and in the future. For me, well into my 20s, dissatisfaction and futility were the ever-present feelings.

Ayurveda's empowerment for me was that it brought me to an

understanding of connection to source, and being made of the same material as the world around me. I realized that giving is the essence and flow of embodied existence: giving well, giving back, giving and receiving is the cycle of life itself. This was a new idea for me, of giving, not for the purpose of getting, but as a way to share the gifts I felt within me—a love of creativity, the ability to care, listen and find worth and value beyond monetary concerns. It has been a great gift in my life to share how Ayurveda has led to a blossoming of the foundational recovery I was graced with through the 12-Step programs. Ayurveda offered me a profound feeling of recognition, being understood at all the different layers of my being, accepting my needs and feeling deserving of having them met as part of a communal well-being. That hole in my soul has been filled by finding my tribe, by being in healthy exchange with people—to see you, relate to you without feeling the need to fix or rescue you.

CHAPTER SUMMARY

The gunas are natural forces that influence the mind: Sattva—calm, clear and content, able to connect with our inner wisdom and allowing it to guide our actions; Rajas—active and stirring up; and Tamas—shadowy, dark and murky. Through this lens, addiction can be understood as incorrect actions based on faulty perception. The gunas also provide a roadmap into the addictive process: from excessive, outward, stimulating Rajas into a downward Tamas spiral. The movement from this perception of a separate ego self (I) toward others who can help (We) is critical in recovery.

SUGGESTED PRACTICE
Breath Awareness[7]

Whenever you feel caught up in the busyness or pressures of the world, take a few moments to simply tune into your breath. The breath is always right here, right now. Sense the body breathing itself. Allow your awareness to follow the natural flow of air and sensation as breath enters and leaves the body. Sensation in the nostrils, sensation in the throat, the gentle rise and release of the abdomen and chest... the body naturally breathing itself. Simply observing sensation as you inhale and exhale through the nostrils. No need to control or change the breathing pattern, just rest your attention on your natural breathing and feel the sensation of the air as it reaches the nostrils, then the throat, and down into the chest and abdomen.

Student Story—The Source of True Freedom

I am a wellness coach and personal trainer who works with people of all ages and wellness levels. I am also in long-term recovery: 30 years with four different 12-Step programs. For me, the real pain of my addictive nature has been about not being able to get out of my own way, re-living and re-creating patterns that ultimately hurt me, over and over again. I come from a biological family riddled with mental illness issues, manic depression, anxiety, schizophrenia and alcoholism, along with vague illnesses, lupus among them. For most of my adult life I've had nondescript health issues which have impacted my energy and attitude, and caused physical distress. I have used therapists, counselors, doctors, shamans, acupuncturists, herbalists, anyone I thought could help me see my way to feeling better mentally and physically.

Starting in about 2010, I experienced an enormous amount of loss: my "one true love," my confidence, three close family members, including my father. I was completely Tamasic, depressed, sick and just lost, with outbreaks of anxiety, aggression and manicness. Mostly, I lost the sense of knowing who I was, and with that came a deterioration of my health and well-being.

There are times in life when just the right thing/person/experience comes along. In Yoga of Recovery, I came to see that I was forgetting my true nature. I had one foot in and one foot out of my life. YoR confirmed what I sensed: that this would eventually lead to disease. I am convinced that I was very near an outbreak of cancer.

The aha moment of transformation for me was learning about the gunas and the Sattvic mindset, the true power in that place. All my life, I've pushed like crazy or I've given up and hidden. Those were my choices. I thought that if I wanted to succeed professionally, I needed to be driven, to force outcomes. This is what we're taught in the USA, to pursue external success, so I know I am not alone.

Sattva is key in my own world view, cultivating self-acceptance and self-knowing. I coach others now with this idea about the source of true free-dom and I have seen lives completely transformed, inside and out, as a result. Both personally and professionally, I have seen what YoR can do for people by seeing and healing the entire person, rather than just treating symptoms. Durga's synthesis sheds light on the addictive nature within all of us—our culture is rampant with addiction—and offers tangible solutions. The principles are clear and accessible, presented with compassion and no judgment.

I have more energy than ever. My moods are more stable and I have hope for my future. The spiritual path seems less confusing. YoR has helped bring me here.

Denise G.

ENDNOTES

1   Frawley, D. (1999) *Yoga & Ayurveda: Self-Healing and Self-Realization.* Twin Lakes, WI: Lotus Press.
    Frawley, D. (1997) *Ayurveda and the Mind: The Healing of Consciousness.* Twin Lakes, WI: Lotus Press.
2   ACA Literature.
3   Svoboda, R. (1997) *Aghora III: The Law of Karma.* Twin Lakes, WI: Lotus Press, p. 16.
4   AA, *Alcoholics Anonymous*, p. 62.
5   Svoboda, *Aghora III*, p. 16.
6   Coates, T.-N. (2015) *Between the World and Me.* New York: Spiegel & Grau, p. 21.
7   The following are original copyrighted works and property of Dr. Richard C. Miller: The iRest Institute BodySensing and BreathSensing. Their use, inclusion and reproduction in this work are granted by license with permission from Dr. Richard C. Miller. Unauthorized reproduction is prohibited. All rights are reserved.

Chapter 4

THE STAGES OF HEALING

YOGA OF RECOVERY WORKS MAINLY from David Frawley's definition of addiction: "Addictions are a [another] form of psychological disorder. They occur from too much Tamas or inertia in the mind. This is often caused by excess Rajas, or mental disturbance, which is compensated for by providing an artificial calm."[1]

In the previous chapter, we saw that Rajas and Tamas are factors of mental disharmony, causing agitation and delusion. They represent projection and illusion (Rajas), and veiling and denial (Tamas)—aspects of the faulty perceptual process at the root of our addictiveness. A main causative factor in addiction is also how these gunas of Rajas and Tamas affect the ego—externalizing and objectifying our sense of self.

I hope the causal chain of disease is becoming clear as we slowly build a picture of addiction from this Vedic perspective. We have disconnection from spirit, over-identification with our mind-body and its sense desires. The ego, our sense of separation, has us experiencing some aspects of our life as a struggle for survival so we are stressed out, feel apart from, and have trouble in relationships. To soothe ourselves, we seek sensual stimulation externally, constantly chasing the highs then feeling depleted by that process.

Having the gunas to describe our inherent psychology is profoundly useful, especially as we feel the effects of our Rajasic lifestyles in a sense of general addictiveness and as more people are diagnosed with mental health issues like anxiety, panic attacks and bipolar disorder.

The Sattvic lifestyle choices offer a cumulative process of reclaiming our wellness. We need to cultivate Sattva in order to meet the "one addiction process"[2] that is alive and well within most of us. Ayurveda's description of who we truly are, the pitfalls and our untapped capacities offers so much empowerment, hope and resilience to counter stress and prevent relapse. It connects us with the potential for contentment, stability, self-trust, serenity and peace. Even more, it holds the promise of all spiritual paths: that we can go beyond suffering.

The teachings of the gunas really landed for me in the way David Frawley describes them; here I am paraphrasing his descriptions from *Ayurveda and the Mind*: Sattva has inward and upward motion. Rajasic therapies work through the qualities of stimulation and energization; they put us into action; hence, Rajas helps break up the qualities of inertia and heaviness that are Tamas. It is often necessary to move from Tamas to Rajas in order to restore Sattva. We progress from denial and addiction to self-motivated action to selfless service to meditation.

THE 12 STEPS AND THE GUNAS

The directions of the gunas of Rajas and Tamas are outward and downward— the out and down of addiction. The direction of Sattva is inward and upward. A phrase commonly used in recovery is that it's an "inside job." The initial stages of recovery demand a certain level of care that may be too restricting at a later stage. Our crimes against wisdom do not resolve with punishment; they need a fair and objective foundational understanding of our inner ability to find our light. They need a safe and disciplined environment in which we can show up and take action to change. While our own light is dimmed under Tamas, or unsteady under Rajas, we benefit from the steady light of trusted people who have traveled similar terrain and can walk with us as we activate and steady ourselves on our healing journey. Community support is essential for most of the healing journey, and even when we are not in need of group support, we show up to be the support for those who do need it. We counter the ripple effects of the disease of our addictive drives with the ripple effects of the solution of communal wisdom and support.

Moment of Clarity

As we saw in the previous chapter, many people who recover from addictions report a "moment of clarity" as the turning point in their life from the path of destruction to the path of recovery. This can be seen as Sattva shining through the Rajas and Tamas, a moment in which we are receptive to the guidance of our inner wise mind, a moment powerful enough to change the course of our lives, leading us to seek and ask for help. While this revelation of Sattva is a life-saving flash of inspiration that shifts our mind in a new direction, it rarely rebalances the entire system or deeply purifies our intellect; hence, ego and sense-mind are still a major factor as we embark on a program of recovery.

THE STAGES OF HEALING

Let's look at the structure of the 12 Steps to see how it follows the healing path suggested by the ancient healing wisdom of Ayurveda and Yoga. To heal, deep-seated patterns of attachment, stagnation and depression must be released. For this, action is indicated: we must break with the past and bring new energy into our life, which can involve many things like a change of job, a move to a new area and modifying our relationships. Here is often where we need an objective witness who can discern when our efforts are coming from a sincere intention to create a more supportive environment and when they may be reaction, distraction and diversion tactics (Rajas) to get us out of actually looking at ourselves by merely changing the external circumstances—often referred to as "pulling a geographic."

We can view the moment of clarity as a glimpse of Sattva, but not enough to fully eliminate the crimes against wisdom. However, it is enough to get us to a 12-Step meeting or an appointment with a counselor.

Taking the First Steps

In 12-Step programs, we face the ABCs of Steps 1–3:

- ▸ Step 1: **Admit** we have a problem.

- ▸ Step 2: **Believe** a higher [healing] power can restore us to clarity.

- ▸ Step 3: **Commit**—make a decision to turn ourselves over to the **care** of this healing power.

The movement of Sattva is inward and upward. We begin with an inner shift that ignites us with the spark of reconnection with Sattva, perhaps just a small inner shift in our perceptual process. Many people actually describe a spiritual experience as a moment where everything changes but nothing changes. The change is an internal shift. We still need help to make these initial shifts or spiritual experiences sustainable in the long term.

Think of the process of recovery to be like a curve looping upwards. From Tamas we have to move into action, Rajas, and then gradually we can feel steadiness and stability arrive as we experience more Sattva. The 12 Steps follow this same healing path. The 12 Steps offer a spiritual solution; it is not simply about the cessation of using/acting out, it can become a path of spiritual awakening/transformation/evolution.

It's a 12-Step Program—Not 2 Steps

The path outlined is not that we first admit we have a problem then go out and preach to or try to solve the problem in other people. There are plenty of people who may attempt a "2-Step" program but it rarely works for anyone involved. Why? Because we need to get into action and clean house, purifying the murkiness of the Tamas in our mind.

Into Action

This stage of the recovery process includes Steps 4 through 9, and the *Big Book of Alcoholics Anonymous* actually calls the chapter that talks about these steps "Into action."[3] There is work that needs to be done—the house-cleaning process which is continuous, initially as Step 4 then ongoing as Step 10. We have this murky mess of our life, and there has to be action taken to work through it, to dig down and find out what's there—to uncover, discover, discard as they say in the 12 Steps. This is the work of the steps, and it is often done with some kind of daily ritual/reminders of the perceptual shift that Steps 1, 2 and 3 established. It is essential that we no longer feel so isolated and separated, so much of the initial work is done in company, which takes the form of meetings, participation through sharing and serving in the fellowship, and one-on-one meetings with our sponsor. This can be understood as the action that breaks up the stuck Tamasic energies and beliefs. If we try to do it on our own, we are setting ourselves up for failure—and if not downright failure, a really rough ride, much harder than it has to be. Stick with the "We"!

Sobriety, Mental Stability and Emotional Maturity

Steps 10 to 12 suggest more Sattvic practices, helping us be aware of our tendency to gravitate again toward an external, feel-good solution. It is so easy to fall into the illusion of believing the fix is external to us and in the future, not present within us: more money, new relationships, the next thing that we are going to buy that will fix the feelings within.

▸ Step 10 is continuing to take self-inventory on a daily basis.

▸ Step 11 is daily prayer and meditation.

▸ Step 12 asks that we carry the message of healing through service to others and practice spiritual principles in all our affairs.

In our chapter on sense acting out you'll see how important this phrase "in all our affairs" is as there is rarely just one "drug/behavior" of choice that we act out with. We need to look at all the affairs our ego/senses continue to be involved with.

The healing path of the 12 Steps clearly mirrors the knowledge of both Yoga and Ayurveda. To shift out of Tamas, we have to get into action, guided by peers who have solved their problem using the steps. Then, to calm our reactivity and ego-sense-mind tendencies we need the internalizing process of daily self-inventory, prayer and meditation, which leads us to responsible and restorative action. These are what help sustain us on our path, increase our emotional sobriety and serenity, and help us evolve and grow spiritually. We haven't come full circle in our healing until we stabilize our Rajasic and Tamasic reactions and resistance with consistent daily Sattvic practices.

This is seldom a straight road; most of us experience a kind of looping journey, where we might fall back down again through a relapse or we hit an emotional bottom in another area of our life, but we recognize our situation more swiftly and spend less and less time down there. At the outset we might fall down more regularly, but that eventually levels out. The more time abstinent, in better company and especially in practicing all 12 Steps, the more stable (Sattvic) we become.

THE COMPANY OF THE WISE AND SOLITUDE

After firmly establishing ourselves in these practices, we come to a point when we can safely go into solitude. Solitude is very different from isolation; however, oftentimes Tamas will try to look like Sattva. In both instances the person is alone, but one person is alone in solitude, because they are strong enough to be in their own company, and the other person is alone because they reject company, they don't want to be seen, they are hiding. There is a big difference between taking some time out on a retreat and locking yourself in the house, full of bitterness or shame and not coming out to play!

The more Sattvic we become, the more we have regular connection with the inner contentment and calm that is our true nature. We'll be able to self-initiate a healthy daily routine and experience a feeling of peace. We take time in our day for silence, solitude and stillness. We develop faith and freedom. These are the gifts of the practices.

To remain balanced in recovery and life in general it's clear we often employ all of the levels of support available to us. There are areas where we need to be compelled to show up, there are other areas where we generally have enough interest but still benefit from the support of like-minded people engaging in the same practice, then gradually we become able to prioritize self-care and spiritual practices as we value health and serenity above all else.

I took a one-month long residential Yoga teacher training course in early recovery to challenge myself to a disciplined daily routine of meditation, chanting, asana and pranayama practice and study of Yoga scriptures. That was over 20 years ago and since then there have been times where my self-initiated practices happen regularly and easefully and there are also times when I need to sign up for a course or series of classes to help me recommit. I am grateful to have the acceptance and knowledge of the ebb and flow of my own commitment to the road less traveled. The general invitation from my culture and society does not feel supportive to a more internal and contemplative existence. I reach out, ask for and accept all the help I need. I very much resonate with and work each day toward having real choice, described in the ACA 12-Steps workbook as "Real choice is a spiritual continuum beginning at denial and leading to self-honesty, humility, wisdom, and finally discernment."[4]

> ▸ Sattva: Self-initiated practices which may involve stillness, silence, solitude, capacity and willingness for selfless action.

▶ Rajas: Supported and welcomed by the group, a feeling of people being there for us and becoming more able to reciprocate that in a more self-responsible, self-full way rather than self-seeking, codependent and manipulative patterns of behavior.

▶ Tamas: Will often need more strict supervision as we tend to easily fall back into isolation with feelings of hopelessness. This is often described as "tough love."

Basically for the nature of the disease of addiction, the 12 Steps have this beautifully balanced way of healing to bring the person out of the Tamasic state by getting out of isolation, in service, attending meetings, working with a sponsor, going through the steps—a lot of support that is needed to release these deeply entrenched grooves of attachment, stagnation and depression.

As the saying goes, it is simple but not easy. Adding Yoga and Ayurveda to our healing practices provides an additional layer of much-needed support.

CHAPTER SUMMARY

The 12-Step programs provide a road map for recovery that tracks with the Ayurvedic understanding of consciousness/psychology. In Ayurveda, we move out of the inertia of Tamas through the action of Rajas and from there into the steady light of Sattva. In the 12 Steps, which many people turn to after a moment of Sattva/clarity in the midst of the Tamas, we see the same movement, the same stages of the recovery process. With the support of others, healing is not only possible; there is a roadmap for how to achieve it.

Honoring these simultaneous needs of supervision, support and self-initiated routines on the journey of healing, maintaining balance and spiritual growth, we'll continue to make suggestions on how to add more physical and personalized additions to the spiritual set of tools offered by 12-Step programs and other recovery pathways.

SUGGESTED PRACTICE
Eye Exercises
Sit in a comfortable position with eyes open, head and neck still, body relaxed.

Picture a clock face in front of you, and then move the eyes about six times for each of the following directions:

Raise your eyes up to 12, hold for a second, then lower the eyes to 6.

Horizontal eye movements—from 9 to 3.

Diagonal movements—2 to 7, and 11 to 4.

Full circles clockwise, as though you are tracing each number on the clock face.

Full circles counter-clockwise.

Palming—rub your palms together to generate heat and gently cup them over your eyes, without pressing. Allow the eyes to relax in complete darkness for a minute or so.

Student Story—It All Made Sense

My text read: "Driving. Smoking. Christmas music playing." It was a text to my coworker on a bright and all-too-sunny Wednesday morning in December of 2017. I was hungover, fueled with anxiety and racing down the freeway to my downtown office. My text was meant as a joke, a way of illustrating a moment that can only be described as pure chaos. I would hopefully slip into work without being noticed. With my almost cold coffee, I raced past the receptionist and into my office to meet my billable hours in an outfit that was far too tight.

This scene is an example of my life before I found Ayurveda. I was demanding that my body perform extreme acts regularly without a second thought. Downing one toxin after another and still wondering why my skin was so dull and my eyes so cloudy. I would tell my mother and sister about the anxiety I was having. I would blame it on my job or my love life. I didn't connect that it could have anything to do with making myself sick from alcohol every night, then asking my body to digest salt, sugar and carbs to counter the hangover that resulted. This would repeat day after day, worse and more extreme on the weekends, before I finally made the decision to remove alcohol from my life in December of 2018.

When I took a weeklong Yoga of Recovery workshop with Durga in May 2019, my mind was blown open. For the first time since becoming sober, it all made sense. All of it! The introduction of Ayurveda to my life gave me a way to understand the root of the imbalance I felt in my body and my mind. Sometimes I think that I had to go through the heaviness of addiction to truly welcome Ayurveda into my life with open arms. And I did just that.

I had a few follow-up consultations with Durga. I read David Frawley's *Yoga and Ayurveda*. I began wanting to tell people about my discovery! "It is the gunas at play! Don't you see?!" But every time I went to unveil my discovery to someone, I would shy away and tell myself that I didn't know it well enough to be able to explain it and do it justice. But I kept wanting to. So I am pursuing professional Ayurveda studies and training and I continue to participate in the YoR community.

I want to be able to share the wealth of Ayurveda knowledge with my friend Sarah who is new in recovery and a dedicated Yogi; with my friend Katy who has dabbled in all sorts of diets with varying success at healthy weight management; with my mother who still relies on small doses of anti-anxiety medication to sleep each night. I want to share the attainable vision of a balanced and harmonious way of living with my 13-year-old son and with my Yoga students. And I want to share Ayurveda with other people in recovery in my community.

Kathryn N.

ENDNOTES

1   Frawley, D. (2001) *Ayurvedic Healing: A Comprehensive Guide* (2nd edn). Twin Lakes, WI: Lotus Press, p. 262.
2   Maté, G. (2010) *In the Realm of Hungry Ghosts: Close Encounters with Addiction*. Berkeley, CA: North Atlantic Books, p. 2.
3   AA, *Alcoholics Anonymous*, p. 72.
4   ACA (2007) *Twelve Steps of Adult Children (Alcoholic/Dysfunctional Families): Workbook*. Torrance, CA: Adult Children of Alcoholics World Service Organization, p. 150.

Chapter 5

OUR ELEMENTAL SELF

A NEW OPERATING SYSTEM

"ARE YOU OUT OF YOUR MIND? Have you taken leave of your senses?" These are questions we ask ourselves, and others may ask us in pure exasperation, as we get into more and more trouble from our "addictiveness." When we are acting out addictive behaviors, we are generally active in the first part of the threefold cause of disease—misuse of the senses.

We operate through our senses. When we "take leave" of them, we are not just out of balance, we are increasingly unable to function normally—which is through harmonious engagement through our senses. The great news is that we can use this knowledge to point us to the surest and quickest approach to being able to embody our recovery: by bringing ourselves back to our senses.

This takes us to the core of the Ayurveda and Yogic understanding of who we are at a mind-body level: manifestations of the five elements: earth, water, fire, air and ether. Each of these elements is not only at play within us; they create us, and the world around us.

One of the most important things we can do to deepen our study of Ayurveda is to begin to observe the natural world. Notice the elements that are present and how they interact with each other. For example, how the heat of the sun dries up the morning dew on grass or puddles from rain showers. How we hang our laundry outside to allow the wind and sunshine to dry them. How food is plump, soft and juicy when fresh and shriveled, rougher and harder when dried. How a frozen ice cube melts back to liquid quickly under the summer sun. How wooden doors can expand with humidity.

Below, we will explore the Ayurveda understanding of the elements in more detail and learn more about how they operate in us, with special consideration of their relationship with the five senses: smell, touch, sound, sight and taste. This approach to creating health and well-being is valuable for everyone. In the context of recovery, it allows us to embody our recovery, create more balance and support natural well-being.

COMING BACK TO OUR SENSES

Each of the five elements is correlated with one of our sense potentials. Early on in my Ayurveda studies, I was asked to reflect on this connection between the five elements (earth, water, fire, air and ether) and the five senses (smell, taste, sight, touch, and sound), and I've been doing it ever since. Spend a moment considering which elements and senses pair together before reading on (see Table 5.1).

As we know, each sense works through a primary sense organ: nose, mouth, eyes, skin and ears. These sensory organs are how we receive the external world; they are the organs of our understanding of the world around us.

Table 5.1 The elements, senses and sense organs

Element	Earth	Water	Fire	Air	Ether
Sense	Smell	Taste	Sight	Touch	Hearing
Sense organ	Nose	Mouth/tongue	Eyes	Skin	Ears

Earth-Smell-Nose

The earth element relates to the sense of smell. This may not seem intuitive at first. The fact is that we can only smell something when it begins to evaporate: tiny particles (earth) are carried on the air and reach our 5 million olfactory cells. Did you know that astronauts can't smell in space due to weightlessness?

We know, too, that much of the taste of food depends on its smell. I am unable to eat certain foods because of how they smell, especially durian fruit which has been described as the most foul-smelling fruit in the world. Its aroma has been compared to raw sewage, rotting flesh and smelly gym socks!

Humans have around 5 million olfactory cells; most dogs have 220 million—they can smell 44 times better than we can. I became more aware of this connection between the earth element and the sense of smell as I walked my dog every day. She would come out of the door and sniff all around the yard, picking up on who had passed through the area during the night and left their scent. I think of it as her checking her Pee-mail!

Water-Taste-Mouth

Water relates to the sense of taste. We need saliva to taste and eat. Science tells us that our physical body is around **60% water**.

I so enjoy the discussion of the senses presented in the beautiful book *A Natural History of the Senses* by Diane Ackerman. Here is how she describes the mouth: "the mouth appears immediately in human embryos. The mouth is more than just the beginning of the long pipeline to the anus: it's the door to the body, the place where we greet the world, the parlor of great risk."[1]

Fire-Sight-Eyes

Fire relates to sight. I love a phrase I heard from the Irish philosopher and poet, John O'Donohue, who tells of how "night steals color." We have beautiful color around us all day and then when night descends it steals all the color away. We only see the color reappear when the sun comes back in the morning. The sun is the major representative of fire on our planet. Our planet earth relies on the sun for heat and light.

Air-Touch-Skin

Air represents the sense of touch. Air is a more subtle element than earth, water and fire. I am reminded of this by a cue we use in Yoga Nidra, as we instruct people to journey with awareness into different body sensations— become aware of the touch of air on our skin. We are in constant touch with our environment through our skin and it offers a deep knowledge of our interaction.

Research reported in *A Natural History of the Senses* by Diane Ackerman shows that premature babies that are massaged gain weight and thrive better than unmassaged babies. Tactile stimulation decreases stress while touch deprivation causes physical and psychological disturbances. Touch seems to be as essential as sunlight.

Ether-Hearing-Ears

Ether connects us with the sense potential of hearing, which comes from vibration. Ether represents space. Yoga says that the sound of AUM (Om) emanates from the most subtle vibration of the universe; that is why it represents all the primordial energy of the world.

The five elements manifest from the most subtle to the most dense: from ether to air to fire to water to earth. Ether is the most subtle of all the elements; it is everywhere. It is the substratum from which all other elements are derived. Everything forms from ether. All the other elements are a densification of ether, of the subtle vibrational aspect of our being—our spirit and thought.

GROSS AND SUBTLE ASPECTS OF OUR BEING

So far we have looked at the five elements in order from the most gross/dense (earth) to the most subtle (ether). Each of these contributes to our biological systems:

▸ Earth—stability, solidity, grounded and endurance.

▸ Water—fluidity, flow, nourishment and strength.

▸ Fire—light, heat, digestion and transformation.

▸ Air—movement, the nervous system, circulation and coordination.

▸ Ether—the spaces in the body, proprioception (awareness of our self in space) and good personal boundaries.

Just taking one word from each element's description can offer a good portrayal of how we'll thrive in recovery—grounded, in flow, transformation, coordination and awareness.

SENSE ORGANS AND MOTOR ORGANS

Each of these senses work through a primary sense organ. These are the nose (sense of smell), mouth/tongue (sense of taste), eyes (sense of sight), skin (sense of touch) and ears (sense of hearing). These sensory organs are receiving the external world; they are the organs of our cognition of the world around us.

Next are the motor organs, the organs of action. This is how we participate and express ourselves in the world.

The sense organs are receptive only, not expressive, whereas the motor organs are expressive only, not receptive (see Table 5.2).

Table 5.2 Organs of perception and organs of action

Element	Earth	Water	Fire	Air	Ether
Sense	Smell	Taste	Sight	Touch	Hearing
Sense organ	Nose	Tongue	Eyes	Skin	Ears
Motor organ	Organs of elimination	Reproductive organs	Feet	Hands	Mouth/ vocal cords

Ether-Hearing-Vocal Cords

To investigate the motor organs I like to begin with the more subtle element, which is ether. Ether relates to sound; the sense organ is the ears. As we speak the sound comes from our mouth which is the motor organ—more specifically the vocal cords. This relates to our capacity for expression.

Air-Touch-Hands

Air relates to the sense of touch. We feel touch on the skin and we touch primarily with our hands. The action of the hands is given as grasping. Diane Ackerman gives a beautiful description of our hands in her book *A Natural History of Love*:

> Our hands, with which we build cities, diaper babies, till fields, caress loved ones, throw spears, discover the mysterious working of our body—our hands teach us about our limits, they connect us to the world. They are bridges between *I* and *Thou*, living and nonliving, friend and foe. Much of our slang uses the hand as a symbol for the whole person... Our hands link us to other lives, and to discoveries; they lead us out of ourselves on the pilgrimage of experience we call life.[2]

Fire-Sight-Feet

Fire relates to sight and the eyes are the sense organ related to fire. The motor organ of the eyes are the feet, relating to our capacity for motion. If you want to see something clearly you get closer to it; hence, the action is to move with your feet towards it. Here is a helpful way to understand the connection. Imagine a short-sighted person at the opticians for an eye test. They are required to stand behind a line at a certain distance away from the chart. From there, they can read the first few lines of the chart but not the smaller letters, which they could read only by taking steps towards the chart. With each step closer, they can see the letters more clearly.

Water-Taste-Reproduction and Earth-Smell-Elimination

Let's look at the next two elements together: water and earth. Together they form mud. Together, they also form the bulk of the substance of the physical body, which is built and maintained by food. In Ayurveda the five elements combine to create the six tastes—sweet, sour, salty, pungent, astringent and bitter. The water and earth elements combine to offer the sweet taste which is the most building and nourishing of all the tastes. Sweet foods are what primarily build the substance of the bodily tissues.

The deepest layer of tissue according to Ayurveda is the reproductive fluids which allow us to procreate, to create life.

There is a Vedic maxim: "Life seeks life." As living beings we need to receive air, water and food to stay alive. The bulk of the large mass of food we ingest becomes the body tissues. It is then refined into the drops of reproductive fluid that allows us to re-create life itself. The motor organ of the water element is the genitals/reproductive organs. The motor organ of the earth element is the anus, the organ of elimination. We eat food, take from it what we need and eliminate what is not needed.

Taming/Restraining Our Senses

We are beginning to build a map of connections between the elements and how they operate within our human mind-body system. We always embark on our work with the physical body in remembrance of our existence at the level of consciousness. Our sense of identity in Yoga and Ayurveda should rest fundamentally in our essential nature as spirit—which is animated through the five elements, senses, sense organs and motor organs: our operating system.

In Ayurveda, we work with the body to influence the mind, and the mind is pacified when the senses are controlled. The motor organs, particularly the speech and reproductive organs, are harder to control than the sense organs; there is more urgency to their expression. Ayurveda brings our attention to our actions in a very sense-able way.

THE CORTICAL HOMUNCULUS[3]

Modern science has provided us with a view of our humanness through the representation of the cortical homunculus. This is a distorted representation of the human body, based on a neurological "map" of the areas and proportions of the human brain dedicated to processing motor functions, or sensory functions, for different parts of the body.

▸ A **motor homunculus** represents a map of brain areas dedicated to *motor* processing for different anatomical divisions of the body.

▸ A **sensory homunculus** represents a map of brain areas dedicated to *sensory* processing for different anatomical divisions of the body.

The amount of cortex devoted to any given body region is not proportional to that body region's surface area or volume, but rather to how richly innervated that region is. Areas of the body with more complex and/or more numerous sensory or motor connections are represented as larger in the homunculus, while those with less complex and/or less numerous connections are represented as smaller. In other words, the five senses and five organs of action have been mapped in terms of their relative real estate in the brain. The resulting image (see Figure 5.1) is that of a distorted human body, with disproportionately huge hands, lips and face.

And in Figure 5.2 is the recently presented female homunculus, sculpted by Haven Wright.

The sensory homunculus visualizes the relative weight/space of the receptors in the brain that receive input from the body. For instance, the lips, hands, feet and sex organs are more sensitive than other parts of the body, so these areas of the brain are assigned more nerve endings in the sensory (incoming) cortex. The sensory homunculus reflects this by having grossly large lips, hands, feet and genitals.

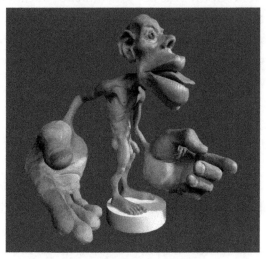

Figure 5.1 Sensory homunculus
Source: NHM Images, Asset ID: 5275

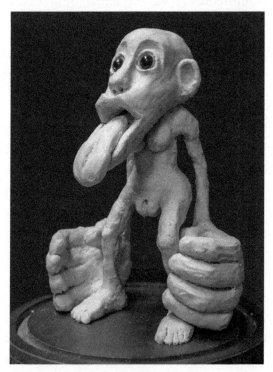

Figure 5.2 The female homunculus sculpted by Haven Wright
Source: © Haven Wright. Photo by Preston Foerder

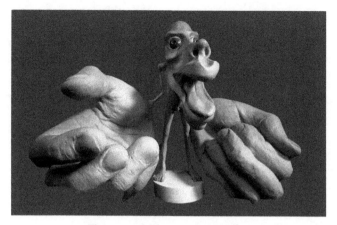

Figure 5.3 Motor Homunculus
Source: NHM Images, Asset ID: 5283

Every body part also has a motor connection in the cerebral cortex. The motor homunculus is comprised of the pathways from the brain that control voluntary movement.

The motor (outgoing) homunculus shows the thumb, which is used in thousands of complex activities, as much larger than the thigh with its relatively simple movement.

When I see the homunculus image, I imagine myself resembling this image when I'm running after gratification at the sense level—frightening! This image really brought home to me the deep intelligence of the Ayurveda system of five elements, five senses, five sense organs and five motor organs. Thousands of years ago, these precise relationships between body and mind were understood—without sophisticated equipment like MRI and PET scans. Neuroscience is now discovering what the ancient healing system of Ayurveda is based on: that each sensation, feeling, emotion, thought and image reflexes to particular parts of the brain.

Isn't it interesting that the homunculus mapping seems to show up in this observation, again from Diane Ackerman:

What is a sense of one's self? To a large extent, it has to do with touch, with how we feel. Our proprioceptors (from Latin for 'one's own' receptors) keep us informed about where we are in space, if our stomachs are busy... where our legs, arms, head are, how we're moving, what we feel like from moment to moment. Not that our sense of self is necessarily accurate. We all have an exaggerated mental picture of our body, with a big head, hands, mouth and genitals, and small trunk; children often draw people with big heads and hands, because that is the way their body feels to them.[4]

OUR NEW SENSE-BASED OPERATING SYSTEM

One aspect of the brilliance of Ayurveda is its recognition that we can work with the body to bring health and balance to the mind. The daily routines of Ayurveda not only provide daily care for the sense organs—they have always been a profound brain science. Proper attention of the physical body through Ayurveda daily routines induces flows of energy within the corollary circuits of the brain.

What we do on a daily basis offers a comprehensive package of self-care for both mind and body, brain and function. I think of this as our new operating system: how we receive the world and express ourselves in the world.

For example, one of the primary aspects of our sense-based being is the air element and the sense of touch, our hands, which occupies a large portion of our brain. Therefore, what we do with our hands has a lot to do with how our brain is affected.

In some ways, this new operating system may not seem new—even as children, we are aware of our five senses. We are generally less aware, however, of our thinking, our cognition; the mind is behind all the senses. Few of us find a way to understand how we can be unconsciously driven by our senses.

The reason that we need to learn how to pay attention to ourselves at the sensory and motor level, and beneath that, at the elemental and sense level, is that the mind's perceptual process is often dominated by the influence of the gunas of Rajas and Tamas. This means that we react to what we are perceiving through a mind that functions under a certain level of illusion, desire, distraction and perhaps delusion. This creates a personal level of distortion of our own sensory apparatus, and our main perceptual process. For instance, slot machines may go unnoticed by those who are uninterested in gambling—but to a gambler, they may trigger excitement and sensory craving.

Connecting with our elemental selves through our new operating system sets us up for creating harmony, health and flourishing in ourselves.

PUTTING THINGS TOGETHER

Operating from our new understandings, we gain a fresh perspective on the sources of our actions, particularly when we are looking at our "addictiveness." Going back to our foundational perspective, remember that Ayurveda says that the first cause of disease is the misuse of the senses, or the unwholesome conjunction of the senses with the objects of their affection. Now we can see how this works.

In a recovery process, consideration of our addictive behaviors through the lens of the misuse of our senses can help us see the particular elements, senses and sensory or motor organs involved. What are we up to with our hands? Feet? The words we speak? The food we choose to eat? Our sexual activity? I invite you to focus on your more problematic behaviors and actions, the ones you are concerned about and want to change.

AMONG THE CHALLENGES

It is important to know that all of the elements and senses are interconnected; for example, we salivate when we smell food. This is the reason why super-markets opt for a bakery department, so we can be tempted by the delicious smell of freshly baked bread, even if it does come from industrially produced dough. The right smell can drive up grocery spending. Realtors also know that if you want to make your home as appealing as possible to buyers, the smell of freshly baked cookies does the trick. Citrus scents, lavender, vanilla, cinnamon and freshly cut grass also rank highly.

Marketing—Temptations and Enticements

Unfortunately, we are intentionally manipulated at the sense level by media and marketing. At the Mind Life Conference on Desire, Craving, and Addiction,[5] it was noted by Thupten Jinpa Langri, a Tibetan Buddhist scholar, former monk, and principal English translator to the Dalai Lama since 1985, that "it's one thing to have discipline to withstand sense appetites but quite another when we have to muster it while facing a constant barrage of temptations and reminders and enticements from the consumer advertising industry."

Rajas—Imagining, Exaggerating, Fantasizing

In that same conference, the Dalai Lama spoke of the role Rajas plays in our sense acting-out/cravings. He said that craving and addiction involve the role of:

> imagining/fantasizing—inappropriate mentation [incorrect attention] which originates from erroneous judgment... We start inappropriate mentation— fantasizing—projection—there is an element of exaggeration. Not just the perception or experience, there is this extra element, where we attribute attractiveness quality far greater than what is justified.

This is illustrated beautifully in *The Tao of Pooh* by Benjamin Hoff, who quotes *Winnie-the-Pooh* written by AA Milne: Christopher Robin asks: "What do you like doing best in the world, Pooh?"

> "Well" said Pooh, "What I like best..." and then he had to stop and think. Because, although Eating Honey was a very good thing to do, there was a moment just before you began to eat it which was better than when you were, but he didn't know what it was called. The honey doesn't taste so good once it is being eaten; the goal doesn't mean so much once it is reached; the reward is not so rewarding once it has been given.[6]

This state of play among the gunas, the elements and our senses, makes me feel more compassion for myself and others around how we often fail in our own best intentions to quit, change, moderate. To become more successful in our attempts, we need to pacify and ground our senses.

In the next chapter let's look at how we act out using our senses and what damage is done through this. In Chapter 7, you will learn simple methods for establishing elemental/sensory balance specifically through Ayurveda daily routines.

CHAPTER SUMMARY

We operate in the world through our five senses and their associated organs of reception and expression. Because we forget our original spiritual nature, we become over-identified with the senses. In our modern world companies take advantage of this powerful distortion, and we are increasingly manipulated at the level of our senses through powerful advertising, encouraging sensory gratification and stimulation, which hooks into a never-ending circuit of desire that cannot be satisfied. The tools of Ayurveda seek to pacify and ground the senses, working with the physical body to create a harmonious balance in the mind. Bringing awareness to the five elements of the natural world, how they operate and their relationship with our physical senses invites us to experience our body-mind environment from a new perspective. In the next chapter we'll be introduced to simple, practical daily routines that help us remember and respect the power and potential we actually have.

SUGGESTED PRACTICE
Five-Element Body Sensing[7]
EARTH

Sitting or lying comfortably with eyes open or closed, be aware of sensation in the nose and the sensation of smelling... Be aware of the body's weight on the chair or mat, and feel into sensations of heaviness and feeling grounded in the body, and the feeling of being safe, secure and trusting yourself... And experience how this acts on the body/mind...

WATER

Be aware of sensation in the mouth and the sensation of tasting... Be aware of the experience of wetness in the mouth. Connect with the actual sensations of the physical body being comprised of 60% water—sensations of flow and strength in the body... And the feeling of being nourished and trusting yourself. Experiencing how this acts on the body/mind...

FIRE

Be aware of the sensation around the eyes—open the eyes for a few seconds and gently gaze at the scene immediately in front of you, then close the eyes and connect with the dark behind the eyelids... Sensations of light then dark. Experiencing how this acts on the body/mind...

AIR

Be aware of the sensation of touch and of sensations upon or inside your skin and the movement of air around and within you. With your eyes closed, raise each hand to the level of your heart with palms facing each other and fingers gently spread. Bring the fingertips to lightly touch each other then draw the palms together in a prayer position. As you inhale use the strength in the arms to press the palms together feeling increased pressure of touch across the entire palm. As you exhale, release the pressure, allowing the fingertips to remain lightly touching with the palms separate. Do this a few times feeling how these movements act on the body/mind...

SPACE

Be aware of the sensation in the ears and any sounds you can hear, while connecting with a feeling of spaciousness inside and all around the body. With your eyes closed, raise your hands to your ears and gently block off each ear with your index finger, resting the other fingers lightly against your face and your thumb lightly on the neck. Inhale through the nostrils while listening to the sound of the breath. Exhale through the nostrils while making a humming sound in the throat, mouth closed. Do this a few times feeling the sensation of sound and vibration and how these act on the body/mind...

Now breathe in and sense into feeling grounded and exhale.

Now breathe in and sense into flow and exhale.

Now breathe in and sense into the process of transformation and exhale.

Now breathe in and sense into coordination and exhale.

Now breathe in and sense into the capacity of awareness and exhale.

When you feel complete, affirm to yourself that you are ready to resume your alert, eyes-open state of consciousness. Then take a deep breath, stretch your body, open your eyes and go about your life.

Student Story—Befriending My Body

In 2013 I finally sought help for my eating disorders through 12-Step recovery and therapy. Over the years, I have struggled with anorexia, bulimia, binge-eating disorder and body dysmorphia. And while recovery and therapy helped me stop the destructive behaviors and address some of the underlying issues, they didn't teach me how to connect with and accept my body. Through Yoga practice, I found some help. I was able to accept my body the way she is, not view her as an enemy. But we weren't friends.

It wasn't until the Yoga of Recovery program that I learned practices to embrace and nurture my body. The first practice was nasya; this simple practice of putting oil in the nasal passages started my journey of nurturing and nourishing my physical body. I then added tongue scraping and oil pulling. These simple ways of caring for my physical form gave me a deeper connection and appreciation.

I now incorporate all of the practices recommended in YoR in my life. I have a healthy, loving relationship with my body. I appreciate all she does. I also see the practices as a way of making amends for the torment I put her through over the years!

Billie C.

ENDNOTES

1   Ackerman, D. (1990) *A Natural History of the Senses*. New York: Random House, p. 143.
2   Ackerman, D. (1990) *A Natural History of Love*. New York: Random House, p. 272.
3   Wikipedia, https://en.wikipedia.org/wiki/Homunculus
4   Ackerman, *A Natural History of the Senses*, p. 95.
5   Mind & Life Dialogue XXVII – Craving, Desire and Addiction. His Holiness the 14th Dalai Lama's Residence, Dharamsala, India, October 28–November 1, 2013.
6   Hoff, B. (1982) *The Tao of Pooh*. New York: Dutton Books.
7   The following are original copyrighted works and property of Dr. Richard C. Miller: The iRest Institute 5 Element Sensing Script. Their use, inclusion and reproduction in this work are granted by license with permission from Dr. Richard C. Miller. Unauthorized reproduction is prohibited. All rights are reserved.

Chapter 6

MISUSE OF THE SENSES AND ADDICTION

NOW THAT WE HAVE A NEW OPERATING SYSTEM, let's take a closer look at addiction through one of the aspects of Ayurveda's threefold cause of disease: misuse of the senses. Of course, as we have seen, this always begins with forgetting our true nature as spirit—and the failure of the intellect, where we can liken the intellect to a gatekeeper who is being bribed by the senses and the objects of the world.

In the chapter on the gunas, we discussed how our Rajasic society is increasingly hyper-sensory and hyper-stimulated. We are seeing the effects of this in our modern "addictiveness." In addition to rampant substance abuse, many people struggle with acting out behaviors, bad habits, self-destructive and self-negating tendencies. In some ways, we are all in recovery from our modern culture.

In his book *In the Realm of Hungry Ghosts*, Gabor Maté gives what I think is one of the best descriptions of addiction as "where we constantly seek something outside ourselves to curb an insatiable yearning for relief or fulfillment."[1] He writes that there is "one addiction process," no matter the expression—"lethal substance dependencies or frantic self-soothing of over-eaters or shopaholics; the obsessions of gamblers, sexaholics, and compulsive Internet users; or the socially acceptable and even admired behaviors of the workaholic."[2]

One of the difficult questions with these habits/behaviors is: "When do they actually become an addiction?" While this is an important inquiry, within a holistic healing system such as Ayurveda, we are able to flag disease-causing factors well in advance of them needing to be termed addiction.

Ayurveda principles and practices can be used in recovery—and also in preventing the highly probable but avoidable compulsive, obsessive or self-defeating behaviors many of us feel plagued by.

PREVENTING CRISIS

At some point, many of us may sense that we are not heading in a good direction but feel unable to stop or moderate our behavior; maybe we do not, or are not yet ready, to consider it an addiction. As we know, the third cause of disease—the effects of time and environment—ensures that disease/addiction will lead to some kind of "bottom": lack of self-esteem, inability to pay bills, job loss, breakups/divorce, diagnosis of disease or condition, DUI (driving under the influence, also known as DWI—driving while intoxicated), court appearances etc.

How can we empower ourselves and others to recognize the adverse consequences at an earlier point? To make practical changes that naturally support positive consequences before we reach a crisis point? In my opinion, it is helpful to end the "them and us" perspective, where we conveniently place the problem of addiction on to the people who have a substance use disorder, the "classic" alcoholic or drug addict, while we absolve ourselves or deny any aspect of our own involvement in Gabor Maté's "one addiction process."

WHAT'S THE DAMAGE? ADDICTIVE BEHAVIORS AND OUR ELEMENTAL-SENSORY SELVES

If we can transcend the Rajas and Tamas in our minds long enough to truly consider the implications of our behaviors, we can begin to fully comprehend our addictiveness and how it is affecting us at the basic elemental, sensory and motor levels of our bodies.

When we consider the root causes of disease, the elemental nature of our being, and how our senses and motor organs are oriented, we can identify a few inevitable outcomes of fundamental imbalances.

This has been very helpful over the years for people studying this part of Yoga of Recovery which is called Between the Mat and the Meeting—Ayurveda for our "addictiveness." To consider what the damage is from our actions—not in any moral or judgmental way, but just looking at actions and their effects. We are not talking, for the most part, about psychological states or weaknesses of character; we're simply assessing the impact. This can be clarifying and illuminating for everyone, and particularly for a person in recovery.

Let us now look at the impact of some of the most common addictive behaviors on our new operating system (in the following chapter, we will introduce specific Ayurvedic daily routines for all of the element-sense systems).

Earth-Smell-Nose-Elimination

Addictions/behaviors that impact this system include:

- snorting drugs

- huffing/sniffing/inhaling solvents

- smoking cigarettes/cannabis/vaping

- over-/under-eating

- overuse of/dependence on laxatives

- sexual addictions.

Snorting cocaine is the quintessential "nose-related" addiction and destroys the health and function of the nose over time, also creating a less and less grounded experience of oneself. Cigarette smoking obviously diminishes the sense of smell—as smokers we don't even realize we smell like an old ashtray! Often one of the first things people notice when they have stopped smoking is how foul it smells.

In addition to its effects on the nose and sense of smell, smoking provides a prime example of the earth-nose-elimination connections. Given our Ayurveda understanding, isn't it interesting how many people say that they cannot have a bowel movement without their morning cigarette?

Ayurveda is not alone in valuing the process of waste elimination in a balanced system. Consider this: while most of us are aware of the opioid crisis in the USA, few are aware that in 2016, a pharmaceutical company launched the drug Movantik (naloxegol) in a Super Bowl ad, where a 30-second spot cost $5 million. The kicker? Movantik was created to tackle *opioid-induced constipation* (OIC). The excessive use of pharmaceutical drugs to induce or replace biological functions also considerably affects our natural earth element system.

Disordered eating, whether eating too much or eating too little, generally results in someone being either too earthbound, through excessive weight gain, or not having enough earth element to support the structure of the physical tissues of the body; cases of osteoporosis, where the bones become fragile or brittle, are common in people with anorexia nervosa.

Water-Taste-Tongue-Reproductive Organs

Addictions/behaviors that impact this system include:

- alcohol

- smoking

- caffeine

- over-/under-eating

- eating disorders—a consequence of which can be amenorrhea (cessation of menses)

- oral fixations

- sexual addictions.

The word for taste in Sanskrit is "Rasa;" it is also the word for emotions. Generally, water also represents the actual physicality of the body; it is said that up to 60% of the human adult body is water.

Smoking diminishes our sense of taste—think about how many people use smoking as an appetite suppressant. Smoking also contributes to dehydration especially in the essential moist mucosal lining of the lungs. Drinking alcohol and coffee also both lead to dehydration, a reduction of water in the body.

Disordered eating, such as eating purely for sense pleasure, the gratification of the tongue, or emotional eating, as a way to replace feeling, causes imbalances in the water-taste-tongue-reproduction system.

Extreme cases of restrictive eating can lead to cessation of menses (amenorrhea), a shutdown of the reproductive function in females.

Sexual addictions can also be understood as a disordered relationship with what are essentially the life-supporting/producing organs, and have an impact in the emotional realms of connection.

Fire-Sight-Eyes-Feet

Addictions/behaviors that impact this system include:

- smoking: cigarettes/vaping and cannabis

- alcohol

- caffeine

- eating disorders:

    - body dysmorphia

    - over-/under-exercise

- excessive screen time

- pornography

- sexual addictions

- erectile dysfunction, more specifically PIED—porn-induced erectile dysfunction.

This is a major category, as there are now so many behaviors around how we use our sense of sight for pleasure and gratification, with so many titillating and tantalizing images on television and in video games. Most people spend too much time on screens, whether it's social media, internet pornography or Netflix binges.

Media images are designed to spark a fire of desire within us, make us see something we want or want to be. Many suffer from disordered eating or body dysmorphia, "seeing" their bodies as other than they are—larger, smaller, permanently flawed or bad, based on some narrow definition of beauty.

Anything that adds too much heat to the body makes an impact here: alcohol, for example, which is also known as fire water. We have all seen the effects of overuse of alcohol, cannabis and other drugs in bloodshot eyes.

Smoking does damage to this system as fire governs the blood and smoking causes blood vessels to constrict or narrow, which limits the amount of blood that flows to our organs. Over time, the constant constriction results in blood vessels that are stiff and less elastic. Constricted blood vessels decrease the amount of oxygen and nutrients our cells receive.

Air-Touch-Skin-Hands

Tactile stimulation reduces stress but many in our society are touch-deprived. Without touch our true isolation is sorely felt. Again Diane Ackerman describes its many purposes beautifully:

> Skin—alive, breathing and excreting, shielding us from harmful rays and microbial attack, metabolizing vitamin D, insulating us from heat and cold, repairing itself when necessary, regulating blood flow, acting as a frame for our sense of touch, aiding us in sexual attraction, defining our individuality, holding all the thick red jams and jellies inside us where they belong.[3]

Addictions/behaviors that impact this system include:

- intravenous drug use

- smoking

- self-harm—cutting

- physical violence/abuse

- excessive tattoos, tanning or cosmetic surgery

- trikotilomania (irresistible urges to pull hair from the scalp, eyebrows, eyelids and other areas of the body)

- lanugo ("skin fur"—a soft, downy hair on arms and legs. This is the body's strategy for protecting itself and creating warmth in response to the heat loss associated with extreme thinness) and other skin signs that are often detectable in severe anorexia nervosa

- formication (the feeling/sensory-tactile hallucination of "bugs" crawling under the skin experienced by those who take stimulant drugs).

Smoking is the habitual addictive behavior that most significantly affects this element-sense system. It is literally the taking in of poisonous air into the lungs, through a handheld delivery system. When someone stops smoking, they often need to plan for what to do with their hands. I know I did. Otherwise I was afraid I would use my hands to deliver more food into my mouth!

My smoking habit started when I was 13 years old. At that same time, I would compulsively split and break the ends of my hair. I'd do it for hours at a time. I often couldn't get my study assignments done as I'd just fritter away precious time splitting hairs. It would help me reach a state of calm and quiet but it drove my mum nuts. "You're like a monkey picking at its fleas," she'd say. I knew it was odd but I could not stop. It was ruining my hair which was so important to me in my teenage years. I wanted sleek, shiny hair (my first Saturday jobs were in hair salons), but I could not stop. Eventually I had to cut my hair short so I could not reach it anymore.

Smoking also prematurely ages skin, changing the skin tone due to lack of oxygen and the 7000+ chemicals in cigarette smoke, and it contributes to skin cancer (as well as lung, throat and mouth cancer).

Ether-Hearing-Ears-Vocal Cords

Addictions/behaviors that impact this system include:

- ▸ verbal abuse, yelling, cursing, arguing

- ▸ smoking

- ▸ disordered eating to silence ourselves—stuff the words down

- ▸ phone sex

- ▸ lying, secrets, gossip

- ▸ self-criticism and judgmental inner dialogue

- ▸ excessive anxiety and negative thinking.

Think about the impact of smoking: the sounds of hacking and coughing; the raspy, rough voice and damage to the throat area and thyroid gland.

Disordered eating appears here in relation to what we are listening to and expressing—What have we heard/been told from the media and our culture? What have we internalized from outside messages, whether from people or systems? What do we say to ourselves? Are we using food to swallow down our emotions? Eating can be a way to temporarily silence or "stuff down" uncomfortable emotions, including anger, fear, sadness, anxiety, loneliness.

IN ALL OUR AFFAIRS—A NOTE
ON CROSS-ADDICTIONS

The English translation of the Sanskrit term relating to the misuse of the senses is "the unwholesome conjunction of the senses with the objects of their affection." We can correlate this to the last phrase of the 12 Steps, "practice these spiritual principles *in all our affairs*."[4] We need to bring the equanimity, balance, harmony and clarity that is Sattva to all the "affairs" of our senses.

It is a regular occurrence that after entering recovery to address a primary "drug of choice," to ease our emotional discomfort we begin to turn to another substance or behavior. Known as addiction transfer or addiction interaction disorder, we replace one addiction with another.

Through an Ayurveda lens, it is quite possible that these "cross-addictions" may actually turn out to be the primary root cause/issues. For instance, disordered eating or workaholism may be at the root of drug addiction where the person has turned to use of amphetamines or cocaine or speed in a bid to maintain low weight or work intensely long hours. It is helpful to bear in mind that often the drug of choice is actually the best "solution" a person can come up with for trying to cope with the underlying pain/problem/distress.

In the next chapter, we will look at Ayurveda's sensible ("sense-able") recovery plan.

CHAPTER SUMMARY

In Ayurveda, misuse of the senses sets off a chicken-and-egg relationship that can be seen as both a root cause and result of addiction. With this perspective, we can see how imbalance in a particular elemental-sensory orientation may directly influence how this fundamental disease gets expressed through habitual attraction to particular substances and/or particular mental states. These addictive habits and choices then create a circuit that takes a toll most directly on the physical body, with psychological and spiritual impact as well. This is why it is essential to embody healing for addiction at the physical level.

SUGGESTED PRACTICE
Scrape the Tongue

This is best done with a smooth U-shaped tongue scraper, usually made of stainless steel or copper. Hold the two ends and scrape from the back to the front of the tongue several times; each time discarding the collected material. Then swish your mouth with clean water and spit out the dirty water.

This routine cleans and freshens the mouth and offers an opportunity to consider the appearance of the tongue coating daily. If the coating is thick, it is better to eat a simple, easy-to-digest diet until it clears up, as the coating is an indicator of the health of the digestive tract and the rest of the body. Ideally, the coating should be easily scraped off, leaving a pink, uniformly shaped tongue with no coating, but it should not appear raw either. If you are not sure what a healthy tongue looks like, most young children still have healthy looking tongues, as long as they don't have colds, are not on pharmaceutical drugs or are not ill. If your tongue is not clean after you scrape it, it is a good idea to check with an Ayurvedic practitioner to learn if there are simple changes you can make to improve your health.

Student Story—No More Relapsing

Yoga of Recovery has been a blessing for me. I first experienced YoR with Durga in 2017. I had been seeking peace, calm and serenity within myself and my environment. At that point, I had been in and out of 12-Step recovery rooms for 14 years. I had practiced Yoga before and was totally enamored by the effect I felt in my mind and body. I did go home and practice some of the Ayurveda methods, but I could not get there, to my peace and well-being. I could not figure out why I was continuing to relapse.

My aha moment came later. In another YoR program, I realized that the "Senses of the Mind" really do dominate our perspective and our decisions for daily living. I began to become more aware of how we should be attuned to them in our everyday life choices.

Now, as I continue to understand and learn about the gunas, doshas and the science behind Ayurveda, I am becoming a healthier individual. I am slowly learning how to apply Ayurveda to my daily life, to not label myself, and am finding my true nature as a human being. Living more in tune with nature has brought me more peace and satisfaction. I am learning to accept my body and that Yoga also is not a fitness trend but a composite practice of mind, body and spirit.

Through YoR, I feel truly loved and cared for, nurtured. I can give to myself and serve others on this path of wholeness.

Laura L.

ENDNOTES

1   Maté, *In the Realm of Hungry Ghosts*, p. 1.
2   ibid., p. 2.
3   Ackerman, *A Natural History of the Senses*, p. 67.
4   AA, *Alcoholics Anonymous*, p. 60; emphasis added.

Chapter 7

AYURVEDIC DAILY ROUTINES

THE SENSE-ABLE SOLUTION

W E HAVE LOOKED AT OUR ACTING OUT BEHAVIORS, the issues we have as a result of the senses having an "obsession" with certain objects of their affection. We are starting to understand how this progressively leads to an imbalance throughout the elemental system of mind-body. Now we turn to a fundamental remedy that Ayurveda offers: daily routines. These are a foundational practice of employing physical techniques to establish a healthier state of mind.

The daily routines of Ayurveda help to develop Sattva in our lives. They provide a manageable way to bring more clarity and harmony to the mind through simple, daily practices. In essence, we take care of the sense gates, and Ayurveda views the senses as the channels of the mind. As we noted in a previous chapter, these sense gates correspond to an abundance of brain receptor sites, so these daily routines constitute considerable daily brain repair and care.

The Western medical model with its current emphasis on the brain disease model of addiction (BDMA) primarily focuses on healing addiction by balancing the chemicals in the brain. Ayurveda and Yoga do this too, aiming to balance the elemental (chemical) forces in the body, whilst also balancing the prana—the vital life force. Prana is more subtle than the chemicals in the brain; we can describe it as an electrical force. The body is described as the Kingdom of Prana and the senses are known as the "gates to the kingdom." They are the gates to our own inner temple of life force. Through the daily routines, we can begin to become loving custodians of the mind-body system.

Yoga teaches that there are 72,000 energy channels (nadis) of prana in the body. Robert Svoboda explains how this number was arrived at: the seven represents the seven sense gates in the head (two ears, two eyes, two nostrils and the mouth), then there are the two below (anus/rectum and urethra), and "thousand" just meant a very large number back in the days of the Vedas (additional gates in women: the nipples and vagina). In other words, the health and vitality of our mind-body system is determined by what comes in, and what goes out of those sense gates.

THE DAILY ROUTINES

Ayurveda's recommended daily self-care routines of the sense and motor organs are ideally practiced every morning upon awakening and as we close the day. They are presented here through the lens of the elements. At the end of each chapter we offer suggested practices to help gently introduce constructive practices and routines into your life. In time, these will become as easy and natural a part of your morning as brushing your teeth. Allow John O'Donohue's words to elevate our daily self-care by feeling into the art of being he describes through a renewed relationship with our senses:

> A renewal, indeed a complete transfiguration of your life, can come through attention to your senses. Your senses are the guides to take you deep into the inner world of your heart… By being attuned to the wisdom of your senses, you will never become an exile in your own life, an outsider lost in an external spiritual place that your will and intellect have constructed.[1]

The Resources section at the back of the book includes suggestions for where to purchase the products you will need for some of the routines. See Table 7.1 for a reminder of the five elements and their related organs of cognition and expression.

Table 7.1 The elements and their related sense and motor organs

Element	Earth	Water	Fire	Air	Ether
Sense	Smell	Taste	Sight	Touch	Hearing
Sense organ	Nose	Tongue	Eyes	Skin	Ears
Motor organ	Elimination organ	Reproductive organs	Feet	Hands	Mouth/ vocal cords

Earth

Walking on the earth barefoot or sitting or lying on the ground are simple and powerful ways to connect with the earth element.

▸ For the nose, we practice **nasya**, an application of oil in the nostrils.

▸ For the organs of elimination, a **regular daily bowel movement** is recommended by Ayurveda. What we eat and drink, our sleep habits and self-care routines all contribute to encouraging this.

Water

▸ **Hydrate**. Drink an adequate amount of water. Also pay attention to your pattern of urination, which should not be excessive or deficient and there should never be any burning or any blood in the urine.

▸ For the mouth/tongue, we practice **tongue scraping** (using a tongue cleaner/scraper) and **oil pulling** (with plain sesame oil or Daily Swish from Banyan Botanicals).

Genitals/reproductive fluids—many postmenopausal women suffer from vaginal and vulvar atrophy symptoms including pain during sexual intercourse, vaginal irritation and dryness. Ayurveda can help with all kinds of feminine health issues; for this it is best to book a consultation with a qualified Ayurveda practitioner. A simple remedy is to drink a cup of aloe vera juice, which is a natural moisturizer. Sesame oil is also a very effective lubricant that can be used locally or on the whole body for Abhyanga (a self-massage with warm oil).

Fire

▸ For the eyes, there are daily **eye exercises** we can practice. We also use special **eye drops** or bathe the eyes with a little Rose Hydrosol (not rose water) in an eye cup. Ghee is also used to bathe and deeply nourish dry eyes.

▸ For the feet, **foot massage** is recommended. This is especially helpful for people who don't sleep well. A foot massage before bed is grounding and can help you sleep more soundly through the night. A nighttime ritual creates regularity and routine that supports the increase of Sattva. You can use Sleep Easy Oil, from Banyan Botanicals, for example. This habit reduces the disturbances in our emotions and psychology.

Air

▶ For the skin, we practice daily self-massage with oil (**Abhyanga**). We take our own hands and apply it to our own skin, the boundary where our inner self meets the world. We participate in beautiful, loving self-care with this self-massage every day and this is profoundly important, as it has a great effect on the nervous system. Science is beginning to show with its research how much touch relates to more subtle aspects of ourselves that are hard to measure, such as pain, emotions and feelings. In Yoga of Recovery, we also consider this as boundary work, using our own hands and touching our own skin, the boundary where our inner self meets the world. Our skin stands between us and the world—no other part of us makes contact with something not us but the skin. (Sometimes dry brushing is more appropriate, for instance, if there is congestion or swelling in the body, and we use very little oil if we suspect there is inflammation in the body.) Again, a consultation with an Ayurveda practitioner can guide us according to our current state of the doshas.

▶ For the hands, we can do **hand exercises** or work with mudras (postures of the hands).

Ether

▶ For the ears, we use **oil in the ears** once or twice a week. Just a drop or two of organic sesame oil or Ear Oil is enough.

▶ For the mouth/vocal cords, daily **gargling** is recommended. This can be done with regular salt water, sea salt or rock salt. Gargling is especially helpful in seasons with viruses, colds or flus as it keeps the throat clear.

These are the foundational daily routines of Ayurveda that create balance and harmony in ourselves through the sense gates of our physical bodies. Through them, we are touching our most elemental selves, promoting well-being in all of our mind-body systems. As you move through the teachings in this book and begin to employ these simple, therapeutic tools, you are actively engaging in an intimate relationship with yourself and the world, cultivating the regenerative forces of life itself.

Simple and Profound

In my own life, there were many times in recovery when I just didn't know what to do to cope with, manage or change how I was feeling. There still are. When this happens, I need to do something to feel better. What I love about the daily sense routines is that they are a quick intervention that allows me to take some positive action in the moment and engage in a more constructive way. The effect is that it brings me back to the present, and I feel more empowered and capable just by taking care of a small detail that contributes to a healthier whole in both the short and the long term.

OUR PERSONAL STORIES—SEEN AS AN ELEMENTAL IMBALANCE

If we were sitting in any recovery meeting together, you would hear about some of my experiences around addiction, and I would hear you share about yours. Like everyone in recovery, I've been through some rough territory.

Step 4 of AA is described as "a course of vigorous action... a personal house cleaning."[2] It suggests a searching and fearless moral inventory. We are to search out "the flaws in our make-up which caused our failure... self, manifested in various ways, was what had defeated us."[3] We've already discussed this aspect of our psychological responses under the gunas of Rajas and Tamas—our ego externalizing and objectifying our sense of self.

The *Big Book of Alcoholics Anonymous* also says "Our liquor was but a symptom. So we had to get down to the causes and conditions."[4] Ayurveda trains its students to treat not just the symptoms but to go deeper to the root cause. Certainly there were emotional and psychological "flaws" that contributed to my "failure" and there were environmental influences—my mother's alcoholism and the general culture we live in. There were also physical illnesses causing emotional and psychological distress, both in myself and my immediate family. The mind affects the body and the body affects the mind.

What I have found useful is to inventory the physical issues that were co-arising with my "addictiveness." As I look at my life through the lens of Ayurveda, the fundamental/elemental distortions become very clear. I can now see how both the physical and the emotional were constantly impacting each other and how I was most often reaching for thoroughly incorrect methods of alleviating both types of distress with substances that had worked, in a limited way, for a short time in the past but were now making matters worse to the point of overwhelm.

I wonder if a look at your own life with the wisdom of Ayurveda will help bring more clarity to the interconnectedness of both the suffering and the health of the mind-body system. I found a **design for living** that involves simple physical practices that relieve my psychological stress. 12-Step programs taught me that it is easier to act my way into right thinking than it is to think my way into right action. Daily self-care is how I act my way into right thinking. These simple physical interventions have had a profoundly balancing effect on my mood and mind. I am often incapable of stopping the useless thoughts that scuttle around in my mind, but I can take positive action to care for the sense gates. As the sense gates are actually the channels of the mind, gradually, with steady certainty, my feelings about life and myself become more manageable. Making the connection between my organs of action and my sense organs and the five elements offered me a manageable, practical, immediate, connected and holistic response to the business of living and relating to everything in my world.

As we reframe the addiction problem and solution in each chapter ahead, I hope you'll see the threads of connection between your own personal story and the component parts of the healing system of Ayurveda. Seeing your own "issues" and life story differently, as part of an interconnected wholeness, will allow you to connect with how even one small change has the capacity to affect your lived experience of your past, present and future.

CHAPTER SUMMARY

Ayurveda daily routines work with the mind through the body, especially the sense gates—where there is a great concentration of brain receptor sites.

These simple and relatively inexpensive practices have a profound effect, increasing Sattva and actually repairing the brain. Taking these supportive actions creates new, health-promoting habits that feel good and can empower a positive sense of self, no matter where we are in the recovery process. As we engage with ourselves from more of a compassionate, self-care perspective, we become less inclined towards temptations of a more self-destructive nature.

SUGGESTED PRACTICE
Gargle with Salt Water Daily

Add half a teaspoon of salt to a cup of warm water (the water should be warm enough to dissolve the salt but not so much that it burns your mouth). Stir until it dissolves completely. Take a big sip of the salt and hold it in your mouth.

Tilt your head back and gargle the salt water in your throat for about 30 seconds and then spit it out.

Repeat the same process until you have finished the whole cup.

Gargling with warm salt water can help to flush out viruses and bacteria, reduce inflammation and pain in the throat, and reduce the risk of developing upper respiratory tract infections.

Student Story—Calming My Brain

My brain has always seemed to run too fast for me, making me wonder if I might be a little crazy. Since I was a little girl, raised with three brothers in an alcoholic home, I have always found myself in some kind of trouble or adventure. I started drinking and smoking pot in high school. The drinking calmed me and my brain down, helped me drown out the chaos. The marijuana made my brain more active—I'd find more projects to do, excitedly get started, not finish, then start a new one. For many, many years I was a combo addict, drinking to calm me down and smoking pot to get high and keep things interesting. My biggest fear was that I was going to miss out on living. For years I moved through different careers to interesting places, meeting all sorts of people, living life "large" in my eyes. It was fun but tiring.

After years of drinking, pot smoking and carrying on, I could no longer keep up. Something had to change. I found the rooms of Alcoholics Anonymous.

I saw that people were changing their lives for the better and seemed happy and free. I wanted that. There was so much of it I liked, but not all of it. I was drinking lots of coffee and eating donuts and cookies to fit in but that didn't feel all that good. I wondered if I was switching one bad habit for another. I knew AA and recovery was my solution, but there was something missing.

When Durga introduced me to Ayurveda and Yoga of Recovery, I didn't get it right away. But her practical way of explaining things and me actually using these ancient practices (alongside my commitment to AA) changed my lifestyle and my thinking. It's the simplicity and routines. My active brain can be calmed! Using prayer and meditation and having a set Ayurveda routine I do daily has trained my mind. Simple things excite and interest me now.

I can finally sleep at night, thanks to the combination of warm milk, ghee and a dash of nutmeg, plus rubbing my feet with warm oil. I can instantly calm myself or change my mood by sipping hot water. I can rub my body with warm oils. Or I go out to nature, where I can listen to the rustle of the wind and the birds chirping, smell the earth. Even if it's for five or ten minutes. Or it could be a Yoga pose. It's the doing that changes things.

Learning about the doshas has helped me understand people better; that we all think and respond differently. We are all just humans wired differently and I have not been crazy all my life. I have found a combination of sweetness in my life through YoR—the combination of the ancient healing practices of Ayurveda with the AA principles of life on life's terms. Both focused on taking things one day at a time, and keeping life simple.

Sheila A.

ENDNOTES

1   O'Donahue, J. (1999) *Anam Cara: Spiritual Wisdom from the Celtic World.* New York: Bantam, p. 58.
2   AA, *Alcoholics Anonymous*, p. 63.
3   ibid., p. 64.
4   ibid.

► Chapter 8 ◄

AYURVEDIC CONSTITUTION

TO THINE OWN SELF BE TRUE—PERSONAL AND UNIQUE CONSTITUTION

Two things really opened Ayurveda as a pathway of recovery and possibility in my life: its view of the cause of disease and its view of each of us having a personal and unique constitution.

Let's look at this Ayurveda concept of constitution. Ayurveda says everything in the universe is a manifestation of the five great elements: earth, water, fire, air and ether. Our own self and everything around us are comprised of the five elements. All of the human differences in shape, skin, hair, eyes, frame, height, weight etc. are due to the predominance of certain elements within us.

These elements combine to form active biological forces within us, known as the three doshas. Air and ether elements form the Vata dosha. Fire contained in water gives us the Pitta dosha. Water contained in earth forms the Kapha dosha.

This was a revelation to me, and it really helped me break through a lot of the veils of misunderstanding and the fog that I lived in. It was important because it spoke to me about a sense of self, and I definitely lacked a proper or healthy sense of self. I was constantly comparing myself with others which was a painful place to be.

Without understanding that we are each a unique organic system, we often attempt to resolve what's going on with us and try to feel better by implementing the diet and exercise principles offered by the "experts" in the scientific media or magazine articles. However, they tend to come from the "one size fits all" schools of wellness. But many of the recommendations may not work well for our particular constitution, or in the current state of imbalance we are experiencing or the stage of life we are in.

If we are following advice and not getting good results, we may tend to think we're lacking in something, and that makes it harder and harder to commit to and sustain these fairly rigorous programs of wellness, diet or lifestyle that we're offered, especially if we still don't feel as energetic and happy as others seem to be.

I had become codependent due to the volatility caused by alcoholism in my childhood home. I took on the voice of the inner critic and always focused on others; hence, I did not have a solid sense of self. I was constantly living with a deep sense of struggle, coming from a place of self-loathing/self-hatred. When we start to accept ourselves, we invite change; the Ayurveda constitution helped me tremendously in this regard.

One of the phrases of 12-Step programs became a breakthrough for me: we are comparing our insides to others' outsides. This concept told me that I wasn't doing well with the one size fits all school of wellness that I was exposed to, consisting mostly of diet and exercise principles. I was asked to strive for a physical identity that I wasn't entirely convinced about or comfortable with, but I didn't know any other way. When I did try one of their recommendations, I couldn't sustain it and it didn't energize me.

Recent data from the Recovery Research Institute shows that we often attempt to stop or change four or five times on our own before we actually admit we have a problem and ask for help. In these initial cessation attempts we go it alone. Often we are trying to find out if we really have a problem, or prove to ourselves that we definitely don't have one! Likelihood is that we don't like the importance the habit has assumed in our life and we fear the direction we may be headed (www.recoveryanswers.org).

TO THINE OWN SELF BE TRUE

What the Ayurveda constitution and the interplay of the elements brought to me was a real enlivening of the phrase "To thine own self be true," from Shakespeare's play *Hamlet*—and also printed on some of the chips given out in 12-Step programs. I was really interested in what that meant. How was I to be true to my own self? Not my crazy, egotistical, addicted, victim self, but my own true self? Ayurveda was such a gift for me to understand myself through the elements and through the doshas. I instantly recognized myself in the description of the air, fire, water traits in my own mind-body. I resonated and related with the idea of each of us having our own personal constitution—it was the first time I ever really felt that I belonged, that I was seen and understood in a natural, non-judgmental way.

Release and Resolve the "Shoulds"

As I brought the Ayurveda perspective into my life, it helped me release and resolve some of the crazy thinking that I had going on. I was able to let go of some of my self-judgment and come to an amount of self-acceptance. A constitutional understanding helped me come to terms with unique personal physical attributes as well as differences in mindset.

As a result, there was a quieting down of "shoulds"—those criticisms from the internal, berating committee inside my head—"I should be less angry... I should be more energetic... I should be more successful." I also held less judgment of others—that same inner critic turned outward—"They should be more considerate... they should be less dramatic... they should not start things and not finish them." These words capture the gift I found in the constitution idea of Ayurveda: "the instant we can accept what is not in our nature, rather than being distracted by all we think we could or should be, then all our inner resources are free to transform us into the particular self we are aching to be."[1] I invite you to find more of yourself in the concept of individual constitution as we continue to explore.

Principles before Personalities

The 12th Tradition of 12-Step programs includes the phrase "principles before personalities," which suggests that the spiritual principle of anonymity of the program is what brings and holds us together. We are asked to practice genuine humility, recognizing and being grateful for our life and our still-functioning faculties. Contemplating the manifestation of such diversity from the five elements humbled me in gratitude for the power of creation that I was a part of. In early recovery, it was common for me to be quickly activated into internal reaction and irritation when someone disrupted a meeting by arriving late, or fidgeted, or was noisy or told me what to do. With the perspectives of the elemental principles of the doshas, I could now see the principles of the function of the elements air, fire and water in the people around me. Instead of taking things personally or feeling superior/inferior, I could step back and observe all of our actions and words from the perspective of the elements in a state of flux. To this day I remain fascinated by the correlation of a person's dosha type (partly discernible from the physical structure of their bodies) with their typical choices and reactions. This is due to the dominance of the elements, influenced by the gunas, so it's dynamic, not set in stone. This was incredibly freeing and allowed me to move toward accomplishing the 12-Step suggestion of the AlAnon program, to detach with love.

Compatibility, Conflict and Codependency

Finally, the idea of constitution also helped me see that sometimes I am compatible with other people or I am drawn to them because of their constitutional proclivities balancing those of my own. Other times I experience difficulties with certain personalities because there's a clash of our tendencies. I believe we've all felt the challenge of this in our lives and it is especially prominent in peer-support groups of all the recovery pathways. We're attempting to show up for ourselves and others. We're struggling with and working on the same character defects (12-Step term) or, put another way, learned behavior or survival skills that are no longer adequate, needed or helpful in the current environment. The trouble is we can often see these traits, what's "wrong," in the other, but we're not always able to see it in ourselves. On top of that it often seems easier to deal with it in the other rather than in ourselves. Remember that this is what Rajas does—it projects the issues and the problems outside of ourselves. This is what I call our tendency toward codependency. The idea of constitution was helpful as it allowed me to reclaim my own behavior and become responsible for it.

HEALTH IS ELEMENTAL

This brings us to a simple statement: health is elemental. The qualities of the five elements can become trustworthy guides on our recovery pathway. We are living in this mind-body system, and we can pay attention and focus on self-care from the standpoint of the Ayurveda qualities. This allows us to take balancing measures as we begin to feel off-kilter, either mentally or physically.

We can recognize our own inherent wisdom, and value our own experience. As sense-based beings, the elements and their qualities are our most innate connection with the world. We know this through our felt sense of our actual lived experience, without even having to intellectualize it. We can balance the life force within us by understanding simple qualities like dry/moist, heavy/light, mobile/stable, cold/hot. This has been our foundation of interaction since the moment we arrived, and truly allows us to live and let live.

Elemental Qualities and the Language of Nature

The ancient sages of India gained their information from direct perception through meditation. They conveyed to us that the five elements display 20 attributes or qualities (ten pairs of opposites). The qualities are the language of nature.

There are four pairs that we focus on in Ayurveda at first because they are quite apparent for most of us. You can think of them like a continuum of:

- ▸ cold to hot

- ▸ wet to dry

- ▸ heavy to light

- ▸ static to mobile.

These qualities also combine and interact with each other, with cold, heavy, wet and static at one end of the spectrum and hot, light, dry and mobile at the other.

Begin to get to know them and identify them within your own felt sense and experience of any physical, mental or emotional symptoms. As you move through the day and through the seasons, you will gain fluency in these qualities of the elements and the various ways they combine and change.

This opens up our dialogue with our world, shifts our perspective and offers an elemental science with a vocabulary that can inform our choices around food, exercise or what the tasks are that we might undertake on a given day or even at a particular time of day.

In case you are curious, the other pairs of qualities are: dense and flowing, gross and subtle, dull and sharp, soft and hard, smooth and rough, and cloudy and clear.

The fundamental premise of Ayurveda is that "like increases like and opposites reduce." If something is overheated, we need to cool it down. Ayurveda teacher Claudia Welch expresses this beautifully when she speaks about the increasing sense of complexity of the developed nations and how in Ayurveda we treat complex with simple. So even when we're dealing with complex problems it's best we keep it simple—the opposite of complexity! Or we could say it's best we keep it elementary, uncomplicated. The 12 Steps also adopt this approach—"Keep it simple" is one of their slogans. Taking a simple, straightforward perspective helps us live well through this one day, and that's good enough; we don't need rocket science! We embark on a simple program of self-awareness and self-care and make use of our inbuilt knowledge to guide us as we learn and grow.

Re-Awakening to the World, Elementally

There was something very welcoming to me; my own self being so deeply connected to the outside world of nature, being made of that same nature. This knowledge—and my lived experience of it—helped me feel much more a part of life and the world around me, less exiled and lost.

I had access to this wisdom when I stopped to notice: of course space is light, ether doesn't have weight. Air is mobile; we cannot see it but we can see it moving the trees. The earth element has a quality of heaviness. Fire is the only element that has inherent heat and water is naturally moist/wet.

The qualities are crucial to understanding Ayurveda medicine and I found the topic to be well within my range of understanding. It wasn't something that I really had to decipher in deep study. It was profound and yet quite apparent.

I began to see that spirit, a divine intelligence as recorded in Ayurveda and Yoga texts, is manifest all around me in diverse and myriad creations through these five elements. Being part of that put me in a more honoring relationship with my own mind-body system, and with everything—and everyone—else around me.

It was tremendously useful for me to understand more clearly that not everybody is having the same personal experience that I am having, quite literally. Even in the same room, even with the same foods, in the same place and time of year, there are differences in our reactions because there are differences in the actual physical structures and metabolic processes that we are each living. All of this really helped me, and I hope it helps you.

THE THREE DOSHAS

Dosha, in Sanskrit, means "that which imbalances." Each of the three doshas operates in particular ways and is associated with a primary site in the body (see Table 8.1). Knowledge of the doshas, their elements and qualities, helps us to find what's off-balance—and suggests a solution to re-establishing balance. We are not a dosha; they function within us. Becoming aware of their tendencies makes us more skillful at keeping an eye on our mind-body system and knowing what is needed to re-establish harmony or adjust to internal and external changes at any given time.

Table 8.1 The three doshas and their elements and qualities

	Element(s)*	Qualities
Vata dosha	Air and ether	Cold, light, dry, mobile
Pitta dosha	Fire and water	Hot, light, oily, unstable
Kapha dosha	Water and earth	Cool,** heavy, moist, stable

* The primary element is first.

** Kapha can sometimes be described as cold; I use cool to distinguish between it and Vata. Vata tends to disperse heat and Kapha to conserve it in the form of tissue.

Back to Basics

One of the main reasons I liked Ayurveda immediately is that it was very sensible. I could easily notice that the five elements and these qualities were at play all around me, constantly changing, increasing and decreasing; it's hotter then it's cooler, it's dry and then it's moist again.

Living with an Ayurveda lens is learning to read the book of life. That has been quite miraculous for me. I didn't need something complex, overly complicated or filled with scientific jargon that I had to have a professional to help me understand—at least not for navigating the daily experience of well-being.

What I needed, in addition to AA, was a way to be empowered in my own embodiment. Ayurveda brought me back to basics and the source of my own knowing. I realized that humans have lived on this planet for thousands of years, so there must be something within us that knows how to live. I just needed to remember it, and to honor and nurture it—that inherent wisdom that lived within me.

My teacher David Frawley suggests that a good way to learn Ayurveda is to simply continuously profile the attributes in ourselves and in our environments, and to see what tendencies toward imbalance exist within them. For instance, I mostly grew up in Scotland where it rains a lot, so much so that the word that is commonly used to describe the Scottish weather, dreich—which means damp, wet, grey weather—was recently named the most iconic Scots word.

I now live in California which is very dry. Water sprinklers were a new sound to my ears. Dryness encourages fire and we are all witness to this consequence with the devastating wildfires California now experiences. If there was more moisture, there would be less fire. To reduce fire, we apply water, and hope the winds don't blow them higher.

This is a very obvious example of our foundational interaction with our world: like increases like and opposites reduce. It doesn't solve California's water and fire issues, but it serves as an example of how we can learn by observing the world around us, the places that we spend our time, and the ways we are influenced by them. As we become more conscious of these potentials for imbalance, they can help guide our personal choices.

The Influence of a Dosha

Once we begin to look around and notice the elements and qualities in the world, we also notice that they are expressed in people, others and ourselves. They show up physically—through both structure and function—as well as psychologically, which we will explore in an upcoming chapter on the gunas and the doshas.

Given these qualities, there are certain tendencies that may indicate which doshic qualities a person most often expresses, a certain approach to life that has implications for their recovery, with specific solutions as a result (we will look at this more deeply in Chapter 14).

▸ A Vata-influenced person—with the primary doshic qualities of cold, light, dry, mobile—tends to use up their energy on multi-tasking, being engaged and busy. Their aim is to do and experience as much as they can and change is often their go-to solution. They may also have a fear of missing out.

▸ Under the influence of Pitta—with its qualities of hot, light, oily, unstable—a person tends to feel challenged by heat. There is a strong competitiveness and intensity, and they can be overly concerned with winning and achieving. Control is often their go-to solution.

▸ When Kapha influences a person, they tend to be a bit more laid back. They may be averse to needed change; even if they recognize the need to change, they may find it hard to implement any changes. They are more inclined to complacency.

TAKE THE CONSTITUTIONAL QUESTIONNAIRE

You will find this questionnaire at the back of this book. You are also welcome to take an online questionnaire—go to yogaofrecovery.com for that one.

I know that everyone enjoys finding out more about themselves and beginning the process of identifying the influence of the doshas in their lives. While it may appear "entertaining" or "diagnostic" at first, ultimately the Ayurveda path leads you to a deeper, more embodied sense of your own innate constitution. This enables you to recognize more quickly and accurately when imbalances occur and the elemental cause of the doshic imbalance that needs to be addressed to support the mind-body in its innate pursuit of health, harmony and positive growth.

In Chapter 11, you will use a Current Life Situation questionnaire to understand the more dynamic aspect of how the doshas are functioning in your life at the present time. We will also come back to the gunas questionnaire to help us identify their influences on our mental/emotional tendencies.

Right now, we are looking at some of the foundational indicators of our primary doshic influences. You will notice that in the questionnaire at the back of this book, the first 26 factors relate to physical structure, which is generally the most stable aspect of ourselves. The next 15 consider physical function and the last 9 describe mental effects. I suggest you focus primarily on the physical structural and physical functional aspects for now.

A Few Notes on Self-Identification

Some people experience anxiety or apprehension around these kinds of self-identification questionnaires. I know I misjudged my constitution initially because it was hard for me to see myself—I didn't know myself very fully as I was always altering how I felt, always comparing myself, judging and berating how I was showing up. In early recovery, our sense of identity can be malleable or too attached to a pathological state. Don't worry. A strictly accurate result is not the goal here. You are beginning an inquiry, deepening your self-awareness. Also know that because of the Rajas and Tamas in the mind, it is sometimes not clear what is our actual inherent physiology and what are the imbalanced states. This can be especially so when we have lived a life of addiction, with rather an excess of Rajas and Tamas influencing our mind.

Be aware that in Ayurveda, we generally tend to treat not so much the constitution, but the imbalance. As we begin to recognize signs of imbalance—through awareness of the elements and qualities—and take steps to resolve our discomfort and symptoms, the sense of self becomes more steady and more clear.

As we bring more balance to our life through sobriety and moderation—physical, emotional and mental—more will be revealed to us about ourselves, even at this foundational constitutional level. Approach this with the openness of simple curiosity; just answer the questions on the constitution questionnaire according to how you've felt throughout your life, the longer term patterns of how you are in life, body and mind.

We will see more questions come up around symptoms when we look at the states of imbalance in Chapter 11. For now, establish an initial comprehension of your general constitution. With many different versions of Ayurveda constitution questionnaires out there in the world, it is likely that you will come up with different "scores" of the three doshas as you take them, as the descriptions are phrased differently or even because you see yourself differently on different days. Again, don't worry; it is the overall proportion that we are interested in.

Remember, We Are Consciousness

While consideration of your Ayurvedic constitution may be new to some, others may have an idea of their constitution or been told something by an Ayurveda doctor or practitioner. What is more important than a label is remembering that we are consciousness and the body is a tool for the expression of that consciousness. Ayurveda states that the primordial cause of disease is forgetting our true nature as consciousness. As a result, we over-identify with the mind-body system, and instead of present-moment awareness, we tend to superimpose the past on our experience of the present with a future that offers more of the same.

In plain English, this means that we claim a fixed identity—I am a Kapha/Vata/Pitta—which is not only inaccurate, it limits our possibilities, keeps us fixed in an idea of ourselves and can encourage us to type others narrowly. Don't get lost in the idea of our identification as a dosha. Be clear that our essential nature is consciousness, our true self. The intelligence of the universe is living through us, through the life force and the five elements. Ayurveda is based in this understanding of an inner self that is our true nature; everything else is a deviation from that.

The human condition comes with the idea of pursuing self-knowledge—not knowledge of the things of the world, but our perception of them. So we'll investigate the way we look at, understand and process the world. We start to inquire about our perceptual process, we work on our attitude because we're not going to change the world, we're going to change our attitude to the world—we're going to change our way of seeing the world, so that it will be more balanced and harmonizing for us.

CHAPTER SUMMARY

Ayurveda provides an empowering, embodied and natural approach to health and recovery, available simply by becoming aware of ourselves and the qualities of the elements internally and in the world around us. We each have a personal constitution, as unique as our own internal experience of life; only we know ourselves from the inside out. Understanding ourselves as consciousness in individual form means we can take things less personally, let go of the need to control, and calm the critical voices that feed codependence and projection. As we study the qualities of the five elements—the language of nature—we see them expressed in human physiology and psychology through the three doshas, the primary indicators of a healthy system and also the primary indicators of imbalance within that system. Ayurveda teaches harmony with nature, simplicity and contentment.

While we may be curious about our innate constitution, and self-identifying questionnaires are fun and useful, ultimately we should not forget the lesson of Chapter 1 regarding the unique perspective of both Ayurveda and Yoga, as well as the approach of 12-Step programs: at our core, we are spirit/ Universal Intelligence. This is stated beautifully by David Frawley:

> Health is not an end in itself... the purpose of physical incarnation is to help develop a higher consciousness... All our human problems arise from lack of true awareness... a failure to understand our place in the universe... The universe rests within us... True awareness is the recognition of unity through which we transcend personal limitations and understand the Self as All... True awareness is the ultimate cure for all psychological disorders.[2]

SUGGESTED PRACTICE

Begin to establish a regular time to go to sleep at night. A consistent sleep schedule will not only help you to fall asleep, it will also support you to wake up feeling rested and ready for the day. It is ideal to be asleep by 10 pm and up before 6 am. If you tend to stay up late, say midnight, shift by 15–30 minutes at a time—going to bed at 11.30 or 11.45 pm and getting up that much earlier too. Make small incremental changes over three to six months.

Student Story—To Thine Own Self Be True

I was 62 years old when I experienced Durga's Yoga of Recovery. I had been sober for three years. I mean, really good and sober, not like the first go-round, nearly 20 years before, when I had gone to a few meetings, counted days, stopped smoking weed and drinking, and figured I was "cured." This time, I worked the program and it worked. I got a major promotion at work that I hadn't even sought and I didn't have a celebratory drink. I went through the traumatic breakup of a very long-term life-partnership, and didn't even think of drinking (though I did binge on a lot of bad TV!). My father died, and I knew how to show up—for my feelings and for my big family. I knew I was in the right place and on the right path. But something was missing.

The two 12-Step programs I participated in seemed custom-made to tend to my mental, emotional and spiritual health. But what about my physical health? I wasn't putting drugs and alcohol into my body, but I sensed that my body itself—the container for the mental, emotional and spiritual being that was "me"—somehow wasn't integrating all the changes that were happening to me.

Enter YoR. Durga laid out the basics for us: these are the gunas, the three aspects of spiritual and psychological nature. Those of us having experienced addiction have been caught in the dark mud of Tamas, and may need to be pulled up by the worldly engagement of Rajas towards the light of Sattva. And here are the three doshas; you will recognize yourself within them: the ether and air of Vata; the fire and water of Pitta; the water and earth of Kapha. Durga systematically drew parallels between aspects of Yoga and Ayurveda on the one hand and components of the 12-Step recovery process on the other. With every teaching, new insights flashed into focus for me.

"To thine own self be true" could be a way of saying, "Know your dosha!" Know your tendencies, your assets and liabilities, your individuality, so you can treat yourself with food, breathing, exercise and other practices appropriate to your dosha, and to the seasons of the year, and for your lifetime. Understand how the gunas are operational in your life at the moment, so you can assess where you are, what you might need, in order to stay balanced, healthy, traveling in ever-unfolding spiritual awakening.

I've since gone deeper with YoR and Durga. As I have continued on the path of recovery, the information and insights I gained from the YoR program have been foundational for me. Even when I am not consciously referencing them, they influence how I think about disease and wellness, addiction and freedom, whether my own or that of someone with whom I may try to share my "experience, strength and hope."

Deborah K.

ENDNOTES

1   Nepo, M. (2000) *The Book of Awakening: Having the Life You Want by Being Present to the Life You Have*. Newburyport, MA: Conari Press, p. 213.
2   Frawley, *Ayurveda and the Mind*, p. 9.

▶ Chapter 9 ◀

GUNAS AND DOSHAS

POTENTIAL, NOT JUST PATHOLOGY

THE ELEMENTAL QUALITIES IN OUR CONSTITUTION show up on a physical structural and functional level, and also on a psychological level. With Sattva, we find the capacity to respond; with Rajas, the tendency to react; and with Tamas, a tendency toward denial, concealment and resistance.

THE MASK OF OUR CONSTITUTION

Mary Thompson, one of my main teachers at the California College of Ayurveda, says that the first mask we put over consciousness is the mask of our constitution. This takes us back to the primordial cause of disease: forgetting our true nature is spirit/consciousness. We mistake our constitutional self for our true self. Our true nature is eternal, not elemental. It helps to bear this in mind so we don't over-identify with the mind-body system. However, 12-Step programs and some other recovery pathways make little or no reference to our physical embodiment, proposing spiritual and psychological solutions divorced from the body. Holistic medicine is so effective because it recognizes the body to be the tangible manifestation of our spiritual and mental/emotional levels of consciousness. Ayurveda is of even greater help as it allows us to *personalize* our care of the body-mind system by identifying the elements dominant within us.

GUNAS MEASURE OUR SPIRITUAL EVOLUTION

In his book *Yoga and Ayurveda*, David Frawley says:

> the doshas are a biological classification that is horizontal in application, with no necessary spiritual implications. A Vata type may be a saint or a sinner, the same is the case with the other two types. The gunas are a spiritual classification that is vertical. It has no necessary physical implications. A saint or a sinner may be Vata, Pitta or Kapha in body.[1]

In other words, the gunas are the measure of our spiritual evolution. Taking this perspective means that we do not equate Kapha to Tamas (even though they share the heavy quality) or Vata to Rajas (even though they share the active/mobile quality) or Pitta to Sattva (even though they share the light/luminous quality). We view the gunas as different levels of consciousness, varying levels of clarity of mind, which affect the doshas (biological forces of the elements) which make up our mind-body system.

Instincts

The effect of Tamas is to be more preoccupied with the body. This can have us operating mainly from a lower level of consciousness: the instinctual drives which are related to survival instinct, territorial instinct, procreation instinct, staying with the herd/being one of the pack, along with a preponderance of focus on our emotions and being very influenced by our past conditioning. Within the *Twelve Steps and Twelve Traditions* book of AA we find such statements as "how instincts can exceed their proper function"[2] and "if we place instincts first we have the cart before the horse; we shall be pulled backward into disillusionment. But when we are willing to face spiritual growth first, then and only then do we have a real chance."[3]

Intellect

The higher operation of Rajas is when we use our capacity for reasoning, albeit unsteadily at first as the intellect starts to become more operational. However, for spiritual evolution it is not the complete answer. The *Twelve Steps and Twelve Traditions* describes this as "Problems of intellectuality and self-sufficiency."[4] As we explore Ayurveda's second cause of disease—misuse of the intellect (crimes against wisdom)—the best examples are the rationalization and justification we discussed in Chapter 3 using the lawyer analogy. At the level of Rajas the intellect can go either way, as Rajas has a dual potential: to lead us in the direction of healing (Sattva), or toward making choices that lead to further harm (Tamas). The AA tells us "our ancient enemy, rationalization, has stepped in and has justified conduct which was really wrong."[5] This again shows why we need the support and guidance of people who are more objective and clear than we are: sponsors, counselors, Yoga therapists, Ayurveda practitioners etc.

Intuition

The more we develop Sattva the more we experience our innate ability to draw forth from intuition, our "knowingness," which comes directly from the light of consciousness; that deep, vast Universal Intelligence that is living us. This statement "we will intuitively know how to handle situations that used to baffle us"[6] appears in the Promises of the AA Big Book. We will be guided by intuition "if we are painstaking about this phase of our development,"[7] which is referring to completion of Steps 1 through 9—the "into action" phase I described as the action of the higher Rajasic force that is needed for us to shift from harming to healing; to shift from the state of Tamas that is addiction.

We see the evolutionary path through the gunas. We can balance the doshas in the body-mind so we can live comfortably within our constitution. Overall, healing comes from developing Sattva—the purification of mind-body—through the higher force of Rajas or the active energy of transformation. Developing Sattva helps to balance the doshas as it activates our clarity of mind so we can be a good custodian of the mind-body. It also gradually allows us to oversee, regulate and mitigate the effects of Rajas and Tamas at our psychological level. The more important and evolutionary process is to establish and increase Sattva, the balance, clarity and integration of the mind. Under a Sattvic mind and lifestyle the doshas naturally come into a greater sense of rhythm and flow.

Self-Knowledge

One of the Sanskrit words used for health in Ayurveda is Svastha, which means "to be established in the self." 12-Step programs use the phrase "to thine own self be true." Knowledge of our Ayurveda constitution can be of great benefit: it can help us to recognize our addictive behaviors and also help us to recognize the actual needs and vulnerabilities that underlie them. We begin to understand ourselves and have command of our mind and our senses. We gain an understanding of the role of the ego, and that helps us become right-sized and more Sattvic.

Ideally recovery isn't ever about withdrawal, isolation or numbing out, which is more of a Tamas state. Nor is it about finding other things to distract us or become overly attached to, which is more of a Rajas state.

UNDERSTANDING CONSTITUTION AND TENDENCIES

While the constitution doesn't, by definition, produce symptoms, it does produce tendencies, and it can produce a tendency towards distorted perspectives because we understand the world from the perspective of our mind-body system. For those dominant in Vata, they may believe that it's normal to have a lot of nervous energy, because that's what they're experiencing. Whereas Pitta may tend to believe that it's quite natural to be intense and driven, because that's how it can feel with a dominance of fire in the system. Kapha people may believe that being passive and sedentary is typical, because they are dominant in qualities of heavy, steady and stable. We can see that these are perspectives created from experiencing the world from a particular mind-body constitutional type.

In his article "Ayurveda: An alternative or complementary medicine?" Robert Svoboda says:

> your constitution is your first reaction to a stress; physical, psychological, pranic and emotional strengths and weaknesses. Your constitution shows your "reaction prints." Understanding your constitution helps you to understand why you do the things you do and what you can do to improve yourself.[8]

Here's a good frame to help understand the psychological tendencies created by the Rajasic mind through the lens of each constitution. I learned it from my work with the Chopra Addiction and Wellness Center[9] and I often use it with clients: "Under stress, I become . . . .":

▸ Vatas generally become more anxious and/or worried.

▶ Pittas generally become more irritable and/or aggressive; they may use sharp language; they may have a tendency to blame.

▶ Kaphas generally need to pause, and it can be quite a pregnant pause. They will tend to get quiet. They're mulling it over; they're processing, slowly.

Take an example of waiting to meet a friend and the friend hasn't shown up. If you're more Vata you might start to get anxious: What's happened to them? You may begin to doubt yourself: Did I get the time or place wrong? Whereas if you're more Pitta, the mind might go more towards feeling irritation: I know we said this place, this time, why hasn't this person shown up? Why aren't they on time? This is a waste of my time, I need to move on. Kapha tends not to be so reactive; they'd be quietly mulling it over. Was it the right day? Do I have the time right? They're not going to react quite as quickly. They'll be okay just waiting. Table 9.1 offers some key words to describe the different reactions of the dosha types under the lower Rajasic force.

Table 9.1 Dosha tendency under Rajas

VATA	PITTA	KAPHA
ANXIETY	ANGER	ATTACHED
Believe that **change** is the solution	Believe that **control** is the solution	Tend to just believe that things are as they are, and they tend to get a little **complacent**
FLIGHT	FIGHT	
		Tend and beFRIEND

Stress Reactions

Science describes a fight or flight reaction to stress. In Yoga of Recovery, we view the Vata activation as more towards fright and flight: remember that Vata is light, mobile and more sensitive, so it makes sense that flight is a survival response for an organism that is dominant in Vata. Whereas Pitta's survival response is aptly described as fight because its qualities are hot, unstable and light. This gives more inner inherent capacity to activate into fight mode. Kapha, with its heavy and stable nature, doesn't have much capacity for flight, nor does it trigger into fight mode, as it tends to have a sweeter nature. They gravitate more towards a "tend and befriend" mode of activation in the stress reaction.

They will appear calm, and they may pacify the people around them, even to the extreme point of "pacifying the predator," but on a more routine basis we can think of it more as just the idea of people pleasing, keeping the peace.

This view of stress reaction is especially important because we are attempting to understand our embodied self through the five elements, the three doshas and the three gunas. Rajas causes the disruption in the organism to an overactivated state which can mobilize any or all of these stress reactions within us. It may be that we are provoked not only according to our dominant dosha type, but also to what the situation allows. For example, as children we did not have the option to leave our homes; we could not just take flight. In many circumstances we cannot resort to either flight or fight. Hence, in many situations the activated states of flight (Vata) or fight (Pitta) reaction may need to be subverted towards keeping the peace/people pleasing—this is still an activated response of Kapha dosha. Kapha is actually representative of our embodied, substantial existence, and it points towards a quite significant biological factor of people pleasing (codependency) in all of us. This is impacted even further as we've lost connection with our inner nature, or essential spiritual self, so we already suffer some level of existential stress due to our belief in separation, which puts us in an almost constant activated state. We live our lives as a struggle for survival, in an ongoing stress mode stemming from our efforts toward self-sufficiency, and using our energy chasing after pleasures and avoiding pain, loss and heartache, all the while fearing the inevitability of death. Without a Sattvic or spiritual perspective on our true nature, we're always going to tend to be more Rajasic—more stressed and struggling in survival mode. Deepak Chopra states this very clearly here:

> this pervasive stress is a unique phenomenon of modern life... Today there's surely less [tiger] terror than in the past but there's more tension, a low to moderate level of background anxiety. For the addict, drugs can provide a chemical antidote to the problem of stress... What began as a voluntary action to achieve a reassuring high becomes a compulsion to avoid a debilitating withdrawal.[10]

Vata, Pitta, Kapha Tendencies

As it is the task of healers to reweave the narrative to facilitate healing it is important to become familiar with the types of sensations, emotions and behavioral traits common when each of the doshas are activated at the Rajas level of consciousness. I offer you this from David Frawley's book, *Yoga and Ayurveda*:

RAJASIC VATA

Ever active, expressive and on the move, striving to achieve various and changing goals in life. Always restless and full of desire, they want to do more and more and can never rest satisfied with anything. They are easily distracted, pursuing novelty and may become hyperactive and inconsistent. Coming on quickly like the wind, they can be overly talkative, superficial, noisy and disruptive.

RAJASIC PITTA

Aim at achievement and success, often regardless of the means or the method. They promote themselves and their agendas with skill and determination, not stopping until they have reached their goal of power and position. They are critical and controlling, prone to anger and intolerance. This leads them to be reckless and vain, which can bring about their downfall.

RAJASIC KAPHA

Aim at acquisition and like to dominate others through controlling material resources. Greedy and materialistic, seeking wealth and position for themselves and their family. Their goal is to accumulate all the good things of life, from home and clothes to property and assets of all types. Driven to own and accumulate and not satisfied until their possessions overwhelm them.[11]

ADDICTIVE TENDENCIES OF THE DOSHAS

Here is Robert Svoboda's take on doshas and addictions from his book *Prakriti*:

Vata people usually become addicted to substances that reduce their pain and insecurity. Pitta people adopt addictions that keep them at the high level of activity that they associate with success. Kapha people often fall into addiction unawares because of poor eating habits that they fail to change.[12]

Vata will tend to be addicted to substances that allow them to keep moving, to keep busy, multi-tasking and on the go. As they start to go out of balance, then they might also seek out substances that calm them, anything that will reduce the pain, anxiety and their tendency to feel insecure and scattered. Vata is prone to addiction; it's advised that they avoid all vices, especially tobacco or sugar and caffeine. These are the more socially acceptable addictions, and Vata is drawn to them, but they are most prone to be quickly addicted to them.

Pitta may seek things that increase intensity and make them feel that they're achieving things faster, more efficiently, more effectively, winning the game. We've said already that Pitta can get controlling. At some point they need to come down from that intensity and feeling driven and then they'll also need to seek out substances and behaviors that help them mellow out and relax.

Kapha is drawn to things that could make them even more sedentary, wallowing in the sentimentality and melancholy of their nature, and also tending to take comfort in food. They are the most likely to be emotional eaters but they are unlikely to recognize this tendency to self-soothe with food as addictive.

Addiction and Consumerism

Within the overall conversation of addiction, a significant impact comes from the consumer society that we live in. This was discussed in the Mind Life Institute Conference, Craving, Desire and Addiction. Many of the world's foremost neuroscientists presented to the Dalai Lama on the brain disease model of addiction. His own translator, Thupten Jinpa Langri, made some very useful points:

> If we narrowly define addiction as a medical pathology then the majority of us will not see the problem within ourselves. If we expand our concept of the psychological mechanisms that underlie addictions, desire and craving—particularly in the context of our consumer society—then we see the critical role of self-control and how challenging that is as we are at the mercy of a powerful advertising industry with very tempting ways to lure us. Simple avoidance is not possible for many of us.[13]

We are considering the psychological mechanisms of desire and craving from the perspective of the gunas. Consumerism actively encourages our addictive drives, and our medical model currently only offers treatment to a few and normally only when the problem is acute, critical or life-threatening. YoR aims to offer help to a wider group of people and offers us a **design for living** that helps us prevent the unmanageability and suffering of excess Rajas and

Tamas; the oft-felt emptiness and despair experienced after we've consumed everything that was advertised and sold to us promising relief or fulfilment.

Both Yoga and Ayurveda tell us the mind is an addictive mechanism. We can bring that awareness into our life without having to "qualify" as an addict within the medical field. The Ayurveda Sattvic lifestyle is both a solution and a prevention strategy available to all of us wherever we are on our continuum of the experience of "addictiveness" within our consumerist society.

RESTLESS, IRRITABLE AND DISCONTENT

The 12-Step program warns us to pay careful attention when we feel restless, irritable and discontent, because at that point, we're probably not going to make the best decision, and the choice that we make could be the choice that leads us in the wrong direction—to relapse or simply continue with our addictiveness in other areas. What is fascinating is that these three words describe the three doshas when activated through the lower Rajasic force: Vata gets restless; Pitta gets irritable; and Kapha feels discontent. Please refer to Table 9.2 for a reminder of the tendencies of the dosha reactions under Rajas.

Most of us are Rajasic, mainly because of our external seeking for happiness, and this can lead to aggression and agitation as it moves to its extremes. Rajas is the mainstay of our active and outgoing culture. We expend our energy on multifarious and trivial choices designed to meet our superficial external sense and ego desires, and this often ends up in a kind of decision fatigue. Rajas brings an over-expression of energy, leading to exhaustion, and this is when the Tamas takes over.

Table 9.2 Rajasic tendencies of the doshas

Rajasic Vata	Rajasic Pitta	Rajasic Kapha
Anxiety, overwhelm, ungroundedness, spaced out, worry, nervousness, rapid shifts of mood.	Anger, aggression, criticism, blame, "hangry", frustration, competitiveness.	Attachment, sentimental, unworthiness, guilt, seeking comfort and ease, wanting things without the hard work.
The colder emotions, and the mobility of the mind from the qualities of Vata—cold, light, dry, mobile.	The qualities of Pitta—hot, light, oily, unstable, so we see more heated emotions.	The heavier emotions from the qualities of Kapha—heavy, slow, stable.

TAMAS AND THE DOSHAS

In Tamas, we become overly attached to the external world of the senses, and we do not pay attention to the inner world of consciousness. When Tamas starts to take hold, there is more danger of severe psychological problems. Tamas can drag us down into ignorance, attachment, emotional clinging and stagnation. In Tamas, we usually choose isolation, not wanting to be around company. Hiding, secrets, lies, guilt, shame—this is the place of Tamas. We are increasingly unable to see, recognize or change our addictive tendencies under our own steam. Generally we need much more strict supervision to be able to make change happen because Tamas describes apathy, inertia, dullness, delusion, denial and depression. Tamas is a lower level of vibration/consciousness where we descend into desperation and despair.

As we have seen, Tamas is the natural progression of excess Rajas, which dissipates energy. This is really important, because our society and most of us living in it are Rajasic; over time we steadily drain our prana/life force, or vital reserves, in this futile attempt to pursue bliss, happiness or fulfilment outside of ourselves. We need to establish consistent self-care and spiritual practices to continually bring us back to remembrance to seek within. The gunas are always interacting and alternating: Rajas and Tamas contributing to our faulty perceptual process that has us believing there's something better out there, in the future, external to us, that we need to get.

DECEPTIVE—DESTRUCTIVE—DEPRESSED

Let's again turn to the descriptions from David Frawley's book, *Yoga and Ayurveda*:

TAMASIC VATA
Deceptive, fearful and erratic behavior that easily becomes extreme, going against any order or courtesy. They are... easily addicted to drugs and other escapes and sometimes suicidal. They cannot be trusted with anything serious and play havoc with all whom they encounter.[14]

Remember that Vata is the air and ether elements, and due to these qualities, we've assigned Vata the stress reaction of flight in Rajas. In Tamas Vata resorts to full escape mode, using substances like drugs or behavioral traits like fantasies. Vata often dissociates from the body. The Tamasic stress of Vata tends toward self-destructive behaviors, for instance cutting, and possible suicidal ideation and attempts. These Tamas effects can occur when the dominant dosha of the constitution is Vata and also when the qualities of the Vata dosha are over-expressing—a result of the inappropriate choices of the lower force of Rajas on the mind.

TAMASIC PITTA

[In Tamas, Pittas become] Destructive and violent in their emotions and behavior. They harbor much hatred, resentment and hostility in life and take it out on anyone who gets in their way. They do not respect any social laws or the feelings of others. Most criminal leaders and underworld figures are of this type. They may be paranoid or psychopathic and should be avoided at all costs.[15]

Remember that Pitta's primary element is fire, and due to these qualities, we've assigned Pitta the stress reaction of fight in Rajas. In Tamas Pitta's natural fire starts to become more aggressive, becoming violent, vengeful and vindictive, capable of bouts of rage. They tend to blame others and can become violent towards themselves and others. In extreme cases, there could be attempts at suicide, or it could even result in homicide as they lash out at another.

TAMASIC KAPHA

Caught in inertia and stagnation which often manifests as various addictions. Their minds are dull and insensitive and they are usually depressed. They refuse to make efforts in life and are incapable of self-reflection, preferring to blame others for their predicaments. They trample over others in their heaviness and lethargy. Their bodies similarly are usually overweight and full of toxins.[16]

With Kapha in Tamas, we see deep passivity, dependency, sleeping too much, lack of drive and motivation. A refusal to make efforts in life, waiting for others to rescue them—this is the unspoken expectation of their people-pleasing. It is common for Tamasic Kaphas to be overly attached and possessive of the people closest to them and this codependency can result in emotional manipulation and smothering of the other. The desire for acquiring things—possessions and the desire for comfort—can lead to stealing and hoarding.

Hospitals, Jails and Institution

If we continue to be ensnared by the lower Rajasic force of our consumer and capitalist culture, if we don't practice spiritual principles in all our affairs, on a daily basis, then that restless, irritable and discontent effect of Rajas will take us to hospitals, jails and institutions (12-Step language) because of the progressive nature of the disease. Hospitals because Vata tends towards self-harm and self-destructive behaviors; jails because Pitta tends to lash out at others, being dismissive of the laws, and deciding themselves what's right and what's wrong; and institutions as Kapha becomes so passive and childlike they may actually no longer be capable of looking after themselves.

Introducing some simple self-care routines and regularity in our schedules are some of the ways we establish more Sattva in our lives. These tools and practices of Ayurveda support our inbuilt capacity for peace, clarity and calm. In the next chapter, we will explore Sattva in more depth, including through the lens of the three doshas. Ultimately, Sattva holds the key to unlocking our full potential.

CHAPTER SUMMARY

The gunas describe the transformative spiritual path; with Sattva guiding our lifestyle choices we have a more sure footing and stability on our recovery journey. An increasingly Sattvic lifestyle is the antidote to the disease process. Our constitution can help to reveal patterns in our stress reaction tendencies. All three biological forces—Vata, Pitta and Kapha—can be expressed through any of the gunas, which represent different levels of clarity/consciousness. Rajas tends to overactivate our biological responses whereas Tamas downregulates them. We move from hyperactivation to hypoactivation. This is the root cause of our chronic lifestyle diseases like metabolic disorder, cardiovascular disease and diabetes. As Rajas is the predominant guna of our culture, and the kingpin in setting off the addictive/disease process that results in Tamas, it is important to consider how it is impacting us and our particular tendencies.

SUGGESTED PRACTICE

Looking back at your answers in the mental constitutional questionnaire, pick one area that was marked in the Tamas column and make changes to shift it into the Rajas then into the Sattva column.

In essence, two of the best ways to shift Tamas are firstly through a simple daily exercise routine like the practice of Asana (a great way to start is by learning a Sun Salutation which can be done each morning upon awakening) or going for a walk; and the second way is offering service to others.

Student Story—Everything Was Not Fine

We planned to meet in Boulder, Colorado, and drive to Utah for a two-week trip with camping, hiking, petroglyphs. It was a big deal. My middle sister and I had been close much of our lives but the last few years had been hard on each of us individually: the dramatic end of my 20-year marriage, her raising a young daughter on limited income. And the past: all the childhood trauma and dysfunction we were each dealing and not dealing with in our own ways. Then, three weeks before the trip, we had a big misunderstanding. Very big. In our family, there are two ways of handling emotional fallout: never talk to the person again or pretend everything is fine.

Everything was not fine. She was hurt and angry. I was hurt and angry. I wanted to cancel the trip. I wanted to make her see how she was at fault. I didn't need her in my life anyway. But I had just been through Durga's Yoga of Recovery program. I had learned so much about how humans function and how life works: the elements, the gunas, the senses, the doshas and how recovery from core imbalances and relational patterns is attainable. I refused to carry on the family legacy. I just didn't know what the other options were.

I suggested via email that we talk in a few days, once our emotions had calmed. I needed the time to sort through it all. On that call, we each took time to speak our truth, to share our perception of what had happened to cause the breakdown. We each had moments when we got triggered but we took responsibility and paused. More importantly, we each had moments when we understood things from the other person's perspective, even if we didn't agree with it. We found new language to describe our feelings and the "facts" that had caused the misunderstanding. We hung up not knowing whether the trip would happen but in agreement that our relationship was more important than who was right or who could have done things better to begin with.

We did meet in Boulder. And we took the trip to Utah together—an amazing experience that we both loved and that brought us closer. I remembered how much I love her, saw more clearly than ever how differently we are wired, and enjoyed how much fun we can have together. Only once did we teeter on the edge of that abyss again. Because, well, the elements, the gunas, the senses, the doshas, childhood trauma and all that. What I know for 100 percent certain is that without the tools and teachings from YoR, we probably wouldn't be speaking now—or ever again.

Grace W.

Student Story—Self-Care Ahas

I had more "aha" moments in Yoga of Recovery than any other course I have ever taken. The self-care tips really changed my life: from tongue scraping, to nasya oil, to foot massages with Pitta oil, to making kitchari again! I started to watch my body heal from a sugar addiction and paused to remind myself I am worth all of these changes and the time they take each day.

When I turned 50 recently, I felt better than ever thanks to YoR. I understand the gunas in a way that they are now part of my consciousness and daily life. I will forever look at the water in a lake differently thanks to the way Durga explained how the gunas function. It has been an amazing experience.

Sue D.

ENDNOTES

1   Frawley, *Yoga and Ayurveda*, p. 46.
2   AA (2002) *Twelve Steps and Twelve Traditions*. New York: Alcoholics Anonymous World Services, p. 6.
3   ibid., p. 114.
4   ibid., p. 5.
5   ibid., p. 94.
6   AA, *Alcoholics Anonymous*, p. 84.
7   ibid., p. 83.

8   Svoboda, R. (2013) "Ayurveda: An alternative or complementary medicine?" https://rare-booksocietyofindia.org/postDetail.php?id=196174216674_10151481805456675

9   www.chopratreatmentcenter.com

10 Chopra, D. (1997) *Overcoming Addictions: The Spiritual Solution.* New York: Harmony, p. 67.

11 Frawley, *Yoga and Ayurveda*, pp. 47–48.

12 Svoboda, R. (1998) *Prakriti: Your Ayurvedic Constitution* (2nd edn). Twin Lakes, WI: Lotus Press, p. 68.

13 Langri, T.J., Mind & Life XXVII: Craving, Desire and Addiction conference, Mind & Life Institute. www.dalailama.com/videos/mind-and-life-xxvii-craving-desire-and-addiction

14 Frawley, *Yoga and Ayurveda*, pp. 47–48.

15 ibid.

16 ibid.

Chapter 10

SATTVA GUNA AND THE DOSHAS

SATTVA

W E HAVE CONSIDERED TAMAS AND RAJAS; now we turn to Sattva, the third guna. The word Sattva is related to the word "Svastha," health, and when we develop Sattva, it affords us a better opportunity to hold our whole system in a healthy balance. The mind-body interaction is so important and so accessible through the perspective of the gunas and how they affect the doshas. We can understand and make more specific use of a range of modalities available to us as we gauge our stress reaction tendencies and apply both activating and calming therapies as required. We can balance action, feeling and being.

In my life, so many areas were out of balance and Ayurveda medicine gave me a simple, cumulative solution encapsulated by the word Svastha, especially in its meaning "to be established in the self." As soon as I turned my attention within—to gauge my own reaction to my lifestyle choices rather than blindly follow more "good advice" from the "experts"—I learned more about myself in just a few months than I had in the previous 30+ years. I recognized my own inherent wisdom and experience as trustworthy guides on my recovery path.

I smile as I share this profound simplicity that health is elemental! We are spirit embodied in an elemental outfit. I can accept and work with the diversity of spirit coming through air, fire or water types—seeing the similarities and honoring the differences, allowing me to live and let live. Many who have learned about the gunas in Yoga of Recovery report a much more dynamic and compassionate understanding of their own mind and emotions and how they can make use of elemental qualities and practices to help balance their whole mind-body system.

The Three Rs of Sattva: Regularity, Routine, Repetition

Unlike Rajas and Tamas, Sattva does not cause disease; it allows the body to come to balance as our choices are guided by a clear mind. In this book, we are aiming to build the ability to navigate out of self-defeating thoughts, emotions and beliefs rather than getting stuck in them. We can begin by achieving significant progress primarily at a functional level, such as being able to get to sleep at night, choosing our food wisely so we can digest what we eat and having regular elimination.

Initially the development of Sattva through Ayurveda wisdom allows us to accept our own identity, as we begin to understand our constitutional self and then learn to manage our stress reactions through consistent action. Recovery is not living in a feeling of deprivation or a continuous struggle to survive each day. It is also not just about letting go of one particular substance or behavior of choice while acting out with others.

Misuse of senses in the outward pursuit of pleasure often reverts to self-indulgence, egotistical selfishness and self-absorption. The solution is that we gradually reveal and stay faithful to our inner wisdom. We engage in practical ways to increase our capacity for self-acceptance and self-esteem. This is well phrased within the 12-Step program of Adult Children of Alcoholics and Dysfunctional Families (ACA): "the goal is self-love and knowing that we are good enough just the way we are. This is an ACA paradox. We do not have to earn self-love, but there is effort in the process of claiming it."[1]

Ayurveda says we can support our clarity and peace of mind through daily physical means. Sattva is developed through the effort of consistent appropriate action. We aim for regularity and routine in our daily schedule through our focus on self-care through simple, practical daily routines. We can work with what we are doing with our senses, what we are drinking and eating, and we can effect change on all layers of our being through the physical. Ayurveda is truly the first and most excellent behavioral health care technology of the planet.

Sattva Is the Balance of Rajas and Tamas

We come home to ourselves through Sattva. Sattva offers us a place of neutrality from which we can see how we have reacted to life. It gives us a grip on our personal reality, allows us to face our darkest moments and emerge knowing we can survive our feelings. Again the ACA Big Red Book speaks to this: we emerge after years of pursuing an "unending number of relationships, schemes, and addictions in an effort to connect with someone who would fix us or let us fix them."[2]

Developing Sattva allows us to sit with uncomfortable feelings that come with life's challenges and adversities. We can pause and consider any situation that's arising; we can ask for help, accept it and follow guidance. Sattva is that ability to direct the inquiry inward, resulting in a clearer, calmer, more harmonious state of mind so better choices are more easily made. We become a good custodian of the mind-body system, able to respond to our needs in a gentle, patient manner.

Sattva gives happiness and contentment of a lasting nature. It develops further as we undertake spiritual practices and we become much less prone to relapse or cross-addiction. I've suggested that Steps 10, 11 and 12 (commonly known as the "maintenance" steps of the 12-Step program) are the steps that most increase Sattva in our lives. We have a new sense of who we are and new ideas of what we need to do. We've gradually gained more mastery of the mind-body system.

The happiness we were looking for outside of ourselves is actually our true nature. Once we draw back from that externalization and futurizing our better days, we can come into the present moment. That's where our search for the holy grail can end. We find the happiness and contentment that we were looking for; it is our very nature.

Sattva and the Doshas

Sattva is spiritual in nature, oriented toward growth and potential. In *Yoga and Ayurveda*, David Frawley describes the ways that Sattva expresses through each of the doshas, reproduced here with his permission and my gratitude. In many ways, these are the ideals we aim for, but under stress and through interpersonal conflict, we can be pulled into Rajas and Tamas.

SATTVIC VATA

Creative, open minded, broad comprehension of diverse topics and quick understanding of many points of view. Excellent communicators with mobile and enthusiastic minds and personalities. Strong sense of human unity, receptive and sensitive to others. Strong healing energy, abundant vitality and are a source of constant inspiration.[3]

This higher ideal of character and our hope for what we'd like to offer into the world is attainable and sustainable. However, without appropriate boundaries and self-care practices then it is very easy for the outside environment to interfere and we just get caught up in the waves—the drama—and become overly sensitive and highly reactive to the Rajasic world of our modern culture.

SATTVIC PITTA

display higher qualities of light, intelligence and warmth, shining like the sun on everyone. They are disciplined, perceptive and discriminating in their thinking, always considering the point of view of others. They are friendly and courageous in their actions with warmth and compassion for all. They function as natural leaders with strong wills for growth and development.[4]

Again, envisage this as our actual ideal and intention, and then imagine the inner frustration that we all feel when somehow we keep getting embroiled in scrapes, struggles, arguments and interpersonal conflicts, i.e. the Rajas effect on our mind, behavior, intentions.

SATTVIC KAPHIC

exhibit Kapha virtues of love, devotion, faith and contentment, which gives them a comforting presence to all who come into contact with them. They have much steadiness, patience, equanimity and balance of mind. They are loyal, forgiving, nurturing and supportive. They view all creatures with the eyes of a caring parent and provider.[5]

Our balanced Kapha nature is like the ultimate Earth Parent/Mother—contentment and constancy are our gifts—but these can get confused and corrupted in Rajas into emotional manipulation or possessiveness to the point that others feel we are overly clinging and smothering.

THE ILLUSION OF SEPARATION

When we are balanced in Sattva, there is less evidence of the ingrained and forceful personalities of the doshic types. It is one of the saddest things that when we experience challenging facets of our personalities, we start to separate even further from each other. Think of how we may withhold sharing with those close to us because we think we pretty much know what their (over)reaction will be (this is our mind projecting, i.e. Rajas)—"Don't tell mom about this because you know how anxious she gets," or "Don't tell dad about this because he'll be so angry and critical." The root of these Rajasic reactions is the stress we experience through our belief in the illusion of separation, and the outcome impels us to separate and, fearing the judgment and reactions of those around us, exile ourselves even further.

HOW SATTVA AND THE DOSHAS CHANGE

Beginning with definitions of Sattva and the doshas as creative, compassionate and contented, see in Table 10.1 how they change from the disturbed, turbulent effect of Rajas and the stagnant, heavy effect of Tamas.

Table 10.1 Gunas and doshas

	Vata	Pitta	Kapha
Sattva	Creative	Compassionate	Contented
	Artistic, healers, enthusiastic, great vitality	Warm, friendly, great teachers, leaders, guides	Loving, kind, devoted, faithful, patient
Rajas	Anxiety	Anger	Attached
Tamas	Deceptive	Destructive	Depressed
12-Step Phrasing:			
Sattva	Happy	Joyous	Free

Sattva: Our Potential

People who have experienced addiction who are now in recovery need to know what the forward movement is. Sattva does not move us beyond suffering. It is likely, especially in early recovery, that we'll still be dealing with imbalances and health complications. Advancing from here, as we maintain a fit spiritual condition, we use our practices to lead us to spiritual growth—rather than constantly draining our energy through over-reacting to the conflict and suffering around all of our life's dramas. Established in our self (Svastha), we move inward and upward, feel stable and steadfast in who we are and our choices. We attain serenity and emotional sobriety.

Sattva can also offer us a philosophical perspective of a place beyond suffering that we can connect with and use as a steady base from which to approach and handle all our life experiences. There will be hurdles and hindrances (from our karmas and the Rajas and Tamas in our minds), but as the saying goes, pain is inevitable, suffering is optional.

Hearing about our potential really helps those on a progressive recovery pathway. In YoR we remind ourselves of this through the phrase, "healing is self-revealing." For too long, the Western disease-based medical model has focused almost solely on pathology, aiming to cure the disease while often overlooking the person and how they are experiencing and meeting the challenges.

In meetings, 12-Steppers share their experience, strength and hope—it helps to share this news of our potential with people we are trying to help, to inspire them and keep them committed. Everyone in recovery has experienced some major problems in the past, some may be experiencing challenges to this day, but we no longer have to act out in our addictiveness.

It seems we too often claim pathological states and labels. The Ayurveda description and validation of how we do experience changing states of mind— the alternating gunas, the analogy of the waves on the lake—helps many of us realize the dynamic nature of mind and how we can always find a way to make changes and be more empowered by our next choice of action.

WIDEN THE WINDOW OF TOLERANCE

Yoga and Ayurveda encourage us to increase Sattva through proper action by applying the energy of Rajas. This conversation of the gunas has been paralleled, by Marlysa Sullivan, to Stephen Porges' work on polyvagal theory. Here are some of the descriptions for Sattva coming from this theory:

▸ We can foster resilience—"widen the window of tolerance."

▸ Sattva is a state of flourishing—we learn to respond and receive life differently.

▸ Greater adaptability—alternate between effort and relaxation.

▶ Learn to hold a positive attitude even in the presence of activation—craving, stress, pain, illness etc.[6]

Self-regulation is dependent on the accuracy to which we interpret and respond to our life experiences. In Yoga, we adopt a philosophical viewpoint that our essential spiritual nature is untouched by the suffering of the transient events of the world. Yoga Nidra is a highly effective practice that allows us to connect with this witness consciousness, and thereby improve our response to suffering. We begin to develop the capacity to pause, discern, then respond rather than react.

SPIRITUAL EVOLUTION

When we are the master of our mind, the doshas are less likely to become imbalanced—unlike the suffering we create with a "Monster Master" mind (under Rajas and Tamas) and its egoistic and sensory tendencies.

Table 10.2 shows how the 12-Step program maps the healing progression of the doshas with the gunas.

Table 10.2 How the 12-Step program describes the healing progression of the doshas with the gunas

	Vata	Pitta	Kapha
Sattva	Happy	Joyous	Free
Rajas	Restless	Irritable	Discontent
Tamas	Hospitals	Jails	Institutions

INNER RESOURCE MEDITATION

Progress is made on the path of life when we can surrender our pain and stop taking it so personally. We can take the view that life is offering us lessons according to our karma. Each situation of suffering is actually presented to us as a way that we can move through it, grow through it. It's not happening *to* us; it's happening *for* us—on the other side of the suffering is the gift of greater self-integration and self-knowledge.

To practice this perspective requires a strong intention. In the first chapter we introduced the Inner Resource meditation that allows us to connect with a felt-sense of a Sattvic place within ourselves that we can return to at any time. We recommend that it be practiced every day until it becomes second nature to pause and connect with the inner sense of power that is the inherent intelligence of consciousness in the universe that is living us. We need to take these pause points as we interact with the Rajas and Tamas in our life circumstances, the people, culture and world around us. Allow your daily practice of the inner resource meditation to allow this to become real for you:

> self-love illuminates our perceptions and we view ourselves and others in a new dimension. We recognize a spectrum that transcends language and trauma. We recognize the light in ourselves and others. We realize that everyone has a heartbeat. Everyone counts and has spiritual gifts.[7]

Laws of the Gunas

Learning about the gunas helped me so much because I finally understood that serenity wasn't a destination I'd just arrive at and be there, happily ever after! Even knowing that, there's still often a part of me that thinks, "When am I going to arrive?" "When am I going to feel good all the time?" When I listen to people, I hear our common misperception: we desire a destination of happiness rather than the process of living through our days happily facing whatever comes our way. We expect perfection and permanence from things which are essentially imperfect and impermanent.

Remember that Rajas is inherently unstable and transitional. We can't stay in Rajas for too long; if we don't move into a more peaceful state of mind, we will numb out and go into couch potato mode, withdrawing into a shadowy unhealthy place. That is why we have to regularly bring in all the different aspects of Ayurveda's daily practices. We are working toward living in a way where we have Sattvic practices available to us across all our activities: what we eat, the times that we do things, how long we do things for and who we do them with. The Three Rs of Sattva: Regularity, Routine and Repetition greatly reduce the amount our prana is drained through decision fatigue—the idea that after making many often pointless or superficial decisions (Rajas), our ability to make additional decisions declines (Tamas). The psychological effects of decision fatigue can vary, potentially leading to difficulty in making the right decisions, impulse buying or other avoidance behaviors.

The gunas are alternating, they have a certain amount of continuity and they are relational.

ALTERNATION AND CONTINUITY

The three gunas are always in dynamic interplay; observe this through the movement of the day and night. Nighttime is Tamas, daytime is Sattva and sunrise and sunset are Rajasic periods. This reinforces our understanding that Rajas represents inherently unstable and transitional energy. That is why we need to establish more Sattva in our life and not keep seeking out Rajas—it is an energy that is not meant to be the mainstay of our lived experience, even though our culture seems to imply that it should be with almost everything that it communicates: the messages to be on the go (busy) and on the get (acquiring), produce more, doubt yourself and be attached to a sense of identity defined by externals.

RELATIONAL

Recovery is progressive and what is Sattvic for us in an initial stage may need to be reviewed a year, two years, five years down the road. For many of us we know there is a difference between what was needed to get us "sober" and what is needed to stay sober, and also what is needed to continue to grow in recovery. A description of Sattva is growing in awareness, and this implies that the longer we are in recovery, more will be revealed. This means that over time we begin to see the deeper causes of our addictive behavior and often we seek out additional levels of help and support as we tackle those aspects of our life. It also invites us to deepen our spiritual practices for real internalization of spiritual qualities and not just outward imitation. Sattva gives us the energy, clarity and courage to continue on a progressive pathway of recovery—we may "abstain" from other substances and/or behaviors that we now identify as problematic, even though that was not apparent in early recovery.

Cultivating a Sattvic Lifestyle

Healing with Sattva occurs through nature and the life force. There are many, many ways to cultivate Sattva in our lives, beginning with daily self-care routines and regularity in our daily schedule. In Ayurveda, it also includes things like herbs, a vegetarian diet and Yoga.

Our aim is to increase our capacity for self-regulation and Sattva. With sobriety and self-care, we evolve to be "happy, joyous and free,"[8] the 12-Steps language that I equate with Sattva. We support ourselves with the tools of our recovery program and Ayurveda. In the most practical sense, we have a number of go-to self-regulation techniques, including meditation, body sensing, breath sensing, inner resource meditation and Yoga Nidra (see Suggested Practice at the end of this chapter).

Additionally, these two underlying concepts are key in the pursuit of Sattva in life:

▸ **Sadhana**: This essentially means taking everyday events and making them a spiritual practice, to bring awareness and gratitude to what we are doing. For instance, when we sit down to eat, we see it as a mindfulness or meditation practice, perhaps saying grace, being quiet, receiving the food with gratitude. All of the Ayurveda self-care routines can be approached as sadhana—self-care as a spiritual practice—embodying the (slightly reworded; emphasis added) third step of the 12-step program—to turn our will and our lives over to the care of God as we *understand God*.[9]

▸ **Satsangha**: This is defined as keeping the company of the wise/wisdom holders and truth seekers, and can also include the like-minded in our lives, those we meet with on our recovery path. As we have seen in earlier chapters, it is the shift from I to We that matters very much in recovery, especially in shifting from our habit of isolation (Tamas).

A final note about food: How we approach our meals is one thing; the regularity of their timing is another. What about what we put on our plates? A healthy vegetarian diet is a key component of an Ayurveda lifestyle, and beyond the scope of this book. There are many books and cookbooks available on the subject. Kate O'Donnell has written several modern cookbooks that include education as well, including *100 Simple Sattvic Recipes: Everyday Ayurveda Cooking for a Calm, Clear Mind*.

CHAPTER SUMMARY

At the functional level, Sattva guna creates health. It brings balance to the body and mind and guides us to the happiness and contentment we seek in life—which is only found within. Sattva reveals our inner wisdom, providing accurate self-reflection. Sattvic states of being are not a free pass from suffering, but move us toward resilience and realization of our growth and potential. We increase our capacity for acceptance of what is, thereby allowing us to depersonalize our suffering and more easily make life-promoting choices. The key to cultivating Sattva is regularity, routine and repetition—of daily choices, spiritual practice and the company we keep. The cultivation of Sattva is not a happily-ever-after destination; it is a path to integrated well-being created step by step every day, supporting the ability to create and sustain positive change.

SUGGESTED PRACTICE

Give yourself the treat of practicing Yoga Nidra—go to www.yogaofrecovery.com where you'll find some practices to choose from, among them a beautiful offering from Colette Carroll: "Recovery Nidra—Meditation for Addiction & Healing." Colette has a channel on YouTube you can subscribe to, and this is also taught live on www.intherooms.com where it is known as 11th Step meditation.

Student Story—A New Language

Like for anyone who has lived a trauma-filled life and is on a journey of recovery, my past is primal and includes a host of unmentionable experiences, an overdose of horrible and humbling stories. Uncanny how the mind chooses the most sordid life events to keep replaying over and over again. The pain of such a life can be immobilizing, framed by remorse, fear, guilt, the well-known shame and brief moments of light followed by the dark side of relapse. For me, over and over again.

But the light beckons and leads to a discovery, Yoga of Recovery, a host of compassionate people, an invite to join them. "We had to make that journey too! You are safe! You made it!" Within this experience, I consciously inhale and extend my exhale; without doubt, this is a new kind of new beginning. I learn the language of YoR; it is a language of self-care. I am soothed by the comfort it brings. I am keenly aware that my life will be completely transformed once I master and fully embrace this new language. My smile is radiant. My inner wisdom whispers; I am in the light now. For sure the lure of shadowland will beckon me from time to time but I am certain that I will never reside in that dark place again. I belong in the light.

I continue my YoR journey equipped with tools that will ensure my wellness and survival. I am empowered. Every day I am encouraged to partake in the sweetness of life. I do. YoR life is good.

Hariyah D.

ENDNOTES

1   ACA (2006) *Adult Children of Alcoholics/Dysfunctional Families.* Lakewood, CA: Adult Children of Alcoholics World Service Organization, p. 438.
2   ibid., p. 434.
3   Frawley, *Yoga and Ayurveda*, p. 47–48.
4   ibid.
5   ibid.
6   Sullivan, M.B., Erb, M., Schmalzl, L., Moonaz, S., Noggle Taylor, J. and Porges, S.W. (2018), "Yoga therapy and polyvagal theory: The convergence of traditional wisdom and contemporary neuroscience for self-regulation and resilience." *Frontiers in Human Neuroscience*, 12: 67. doi: 10.3389/fnhum.2018.00067.
7   ACA, *Adult Children of Alcoholics/Dysfunctional Families*, p. 438.
8   AA, *Alcoholics Anonymous*, p. 133.
9   ibid., p. 59.

► Chapter 11 ◄

STATE OF IMBALANCE

SYMPTOMATIC CONCERNS

Now that we've had an introduction to the gunas and doshas and their elemental nature, it is helpful to take time to notice how they are at play in our life. Knowledge of our constitution and ongoing inquiry into how this contributes to our own particular "stress-signature" helps us identify what pacifies us and what aggravates that within us. As we bring Ayurveda into our daily life and recovery, we become more able to care for ourselves and balance our life force through understanding simple qualities of dry/moist, heavy/light, mobile/stable and cold/hot.

CONSTITUTION (PRAKRUTI) AND
STATE OF IMBALANCE (VIKRUTI)

As we know, the doshas are the biological forces of the five elements. When balanced, the doshas support our tissues and bodily functions. When they are out of balance, they cause disease. In essence, diseases are aggravated doshas.

The root of the word dosha is "dush," which means "to spoil." Dosha means "what darkens, spoils, decays." This is one reason that we don't want to overly associate our identity with the doshas—it is better to remember our true nature as spirit, the essential, blissful, all-knowing intelligence.

Prakruti is our basic constitution, determined at conception. Our constitution is the inherent balance of the doshas in our body and is unique to our own body-mind environment. It determines the physical and structural characteristics of our body and internal physiological tendencies like metabolism.

There are an infinite number of permutations and combinations. No two people are the same.

I like how Robert Svoboda speaks about this in "Ayurveda: An alternative or complementary medicine?"

> Each living body hosts a wide variety of strongly-held metabolic patterns which influence its ability to build up new patterns. Ayurveda classifies each of these many metabolic patterns into one of three classes. Each of these classes forms a metapattern, a pattern which actively reproduces itself whenever it is given the opportunity to do so. These three metapatterns are the *three doshas*, the body's so-called "humors." They are called *doshas* ("mistakes," in Sanskrit) because when they are deranged they induce the organism to go off balance, in predictable ways.

> Students of Ayurveda work with the reality of life from the dosha perspective because of its practical utility in everyday practice. The dosha approach allows associations to be detected between seemingly unconnected causative pathways and manifested symptoms.[1]

This idea of the metapatterns takes into account that every individual has psychological, pranic and emotional strengths and weaknesses. When taken together, these form a set of reaction prints, which are characteristic of their owners—much like a fingerprint is.

We all have a unique constitution. The aggregate of these unique properties forms our constitution, called Prakruti. It's the temperament which impacts our predisposition to health, our sensitivity to illness and our response to therapies.

The Mona Lisa

Imagine the image of the Mona Lisa. It is a masterpiece, a unique, one-of-a-kind, invaluable treasure. We are all born as the Mona Lisa: unique, invaluable, created by a master. Our innate constitution is uniquely ours, and will cause tendencies in us, but not necessarily imbalance.

Now picture a sheet of translucent paper over the Mona Lisa. There she is, but now slightly obscured. This is what she looks like when one of the doshas goes out of balance. When a second dosha goes out of balance, add another sheet of translucent paper. Now she is even more obscured. When all three doshas are imbalanced—three sheets of paper cover her—we can't see her very clearly at all.

Vikruti is the Sanskrit word for the current state of imbalance in a person's mind-body system. Most of us are imbalanced in some way—this can be a simple distortion that stems from our life history, or it can be a fully manifested and identified disease. It is the Vikruti we treat—we address the imbalance while taking into the account the underlying constitution, Prakruti. We also include other factors such as age, season, climate, occupation etc.

Think of treatment to be like a restoration of a priceless artwork, like the Mona Lisa. It would be unwise to take a wire brush and turpentine and scrub away at it—as that is likely to damage the work of art that lies underneath the layers of grime. Instead Ayurveda proceeds in a gentler manner but achieves profound results gradually. It is important to consider how pleasant or painful it is to undergo therapy and also if the aim is only to eradicate the symptoms or bring about a deeper change, an improvement and empowerment.

Ayurveda, as the sister science of Yoga, aims to utilize our capacity to balance our physical system by educating about the mind-body interdependence and how this all emanates from a creative, unlimited source. This multilayered perspective provides practicality and promise for those of us who wonder if we have the grit and resilience to be able to cope with the demands of a life that seems to require constant struggle and super-human willpower. This science of life offers us healing at a level that is "Self" revealing—a transformation, achieving a state that is better or higher than our original state. Given the description of the cause of disease and our current view that adverse childhood experiences (ACE) and trauma contribute greatly to the manifestation of our addictiveness it is clear that we need not so much a cure but a positive reorientation to ourselves and how to live our life.

When we have been dealing with imbalance for many years, it may be difficult for us to clearly see our constitution. Remember, Sattva is revealing, whereas Rajas is distorting and Tamas is veiling. In the 12 Steps, we use the phrase: "More will be revealed." As we go into these daily and seasonal routines, we begin to look after ourselves. After a time, we'll be able to notice and receive the gift of our embodied presence, maintaining balance more easily the more we connect with the idea that we are one of many masterpieces of creation.

Creating Health

The very important idea here is that we can make use of Ayurveda to work with the constitution we are living in and experiencing. This is a huge advance compared to a one size fits all approach. Once we have stopped use of harmful substances and stopped engaging in harmful behaviors, we achieve a certain amount of rebalancing of our system. We can then manage our mind-body system, one day at a time, to actively create health and wellness.

To help us focus our attention to key interconnected functions, Ayurveda offers the idea of three pillars of life:

▶ **Food**: Appetite, digestion, elimination.

▶ **Sleep**: Ability to sleep and have energy.

▶ **Relational health**: This third pillar is often named as proper management of sexual energy.

Eating, sleeping and procreating are essential to life. In YoR we like to widen our consideration to our overall relational health—our energy expenditure/contribution and returns/rewards from our physical and psychological interdependence, especially as we understand that loneliness can be as damaging to health as smoking and more harmful than obesity! We extend the ability to procreate to include our ability to be creative and live a life of purpose and service, connected with others—family, friends, partner/spouse, co-workers and community.

It is important to pay attention to and develop self-care routines around these pillars of life: digestion in particular, as most imbalances begin in the digestive system. Ayurveda will help us become able to recognize the signs and symptoms of the different doshas and guide us to make more balancing choices.

Please note that we are not to manage our medical care entirely on our own; we must visit with our trusted MDs and holistic practitioners to do our regular check-ups.

VIKRUTI QUESTIONNAIRE

Hopefully the constitutional questionnaire allowed us to come to an initial understanding of our constitution. Now we are going to assess our current life situation to gauge our current state of imbalance. I like to use the ones developed by Banyan Botanicals; please visit www.yogaofrecovery.com to take the questionnaire and ascertain which dosha(s) is causing your symptoms along with some suggestions to move back into balance.

Self-Diagnosis: Your Digestive Tract

We gain a better capacity for resilience and flexibility as a result of taking the time to get to know our own unique mind-body system (how the gunas affect the doshas). We also gain the ability to have simple practical checks on our mind-body system through attention to the qualities of the doshas (Vata being dry, Pitta being hot and Kapha being heavy). Now we'll introduce their main sites in the body so we can pay even more focused attention to help bring us to/maintain balance. Keep in mind the basic principle of management: like increases like and opposites reduce.

The doshas not only have primary qualities but also a primary site of accumulation in the body:

▸ Vata: Large intestine/colon.

▸ Pitta: Small intestine.

▸ Kapha: Stomach.

Notice that these are all organs along the gastro-intestinal (GI) tract. The dosha's qualities naturally express and peak at these sites, then alleviate. Imbalance begins when the quality does not alleviate, but instead continues to stay high and build up. One or more of the dosha's qualities can be over-expressing. If we can develop awareness and catch the imbalance at its primary site, we can head off further imbalance. By paying attention we can begin to be able to chart and keep on course, maintaining a comfortable level of balance and ease through common sense awareness—adjusting for small deviations rather than either over-reacting or ignoring and allowing the symptoms to worsen.

▸ Disturbed Vata produces gas in the colon causing flatulence and we may feel bloated, with some possible pain in the abdominal area along with constipation.

▸ Disturbed Pitta produces acids causing heartburn, gastric reflux and possible loose bowel movements or diarrhea.

▸ Disturbed Kapha produces phlegm causing feelings of heaviness or sluggishness with slow digestion and elimination which may be slimy, sticky or mucousy.

Signs of Imbalance

Imbalance occurs when an organism is unable to adapt to its external or internal environment. Vikruti is the nature of the imbalance, the current or temporary state of the doshas. Healing is the process of returning the Vikruti to Prakruti. Often it is the dominant dosha that becomes imbalanced.

▸ Vata can become imbalanced due to our fast-paced lifestyle.

▸ Pitta can become disturbed by our competitive lifestyle.

▸ Kapha is disturbed by a sedentary lifestyle and over-eating.

It is important to remember the elements, senses and four dominant qualities associated with each dosha (see Table 11.1).

Table 11.1 The elements, senses and four dominant qualities associated with each dosha

	Elements	Qualities	Sense
Vata	Air and ether	Cold, light, dry, mobile	Touch and hearing/sound
Pitta	Fire and water	Hot, light, oily, unstable	Sight
Kapha	Water and earth	Cool, heavy, moist, stable	Taste and smell

SIGNS OF VATA IMBALANCE

We may experience any of the following: feeling cold, tremors, dizziness, incoherent speech, emaciation, confusion and depression.

There can be excess mobility/hyperactivity at the expense of the vital fluids. The primary symptoms of this are pain and sensory disorientation.

Symptoms of Vata imbalance:

▸ variable appetite

▸ variable digestive ability causing gas and constipation; possible alternating constipation and diarrhea

▸ elimination—stools can be hard, difficult to eliminate with straining and feeling incomplete

▸ sleep—prone to insomnia, difficult to stay asleep, awakens easily and may find it difficult to return to sleep, mind racing, body restless

▸ temperature—feels cold easily

▸ skin—dry, rough

▸ sweats less than Pitta or Kapha

▸ menstrual cycle—may miss periods, flow scant and light.

SIGNS OF PITTA IMBALANCE

Pitta governs the small intestine and its symptoms relate to excess heat. It is worth noting that systemic inflammation, a sign of Pitta imbalance, is now understood to be at the root of many chronic diseases.

Symptoms of Pitta imbalance:

▸ strong appetite, feels hungry regularly

▸ strong digestion, with fire roaring it can cause hyperacidity, burning indigestion, loose stools

▸ elimination—loose stools more frequently, possible diarrhea, green or yellow color of stool shows possible liver and gallbladder imbalances

▸ sleep—light, may have difficulty getting to sleep; awakens easily, falls back to sleep easily

▸ temperature—feels warm

▸ skin—oily, ruddy complexion, possible rashes, hives or acne

▸ sweat—more profuse with a stronger odor

▸ menstrual cycle—regular cycle, possible heavy flow with greater diarrhea during menses.

SIGNS OF KAPHA IMBALANCE

Kapha goes more toward hypo-activity. The earth and water create congestion and heaviness, a lack of flow.

Symptoms of Kapha imbalance:

▸ appetite—slow but steady/constant

▸ digestion—low fire slows metabolism, feels sluggish, sleepy, heavy after eating

▸ elimination—regular; stools can be large/bulky, pale, with mucous; possible constipation—stool may feel slimy or sticky, not hard and dry like Vata-type constipation

▸ sleep—heavy, sound, falls asleep quickly; finds it difficult to awaken/ get out of bed

▸ temperature—cool but not cold

▸ skin—thick, soft, smooth, may feel clammy

▸ sweat—profuse, but does not have a sharp odor

▸ menstrual cycle—regular, flow is average to heavy with greater swelling prior to period.

BALANCING VATA

Ayurveda's ancient texts tell us that Vata causes four times as many diseases as Kapha and twice as many as Pitta. This is due to the mobility of the Vata energy. By learning to balance Vata, we do ourselves a great service. It is similar to knowing how to move toward Sattva, because a healthy mind is the best disease prevention strategy as it holds the doshas at an integrated level of healthy function. First we increase Sattva, then we undertake the management of metabolism (see Chapter 13) and hopefully the management of Vata. If we can treat the doshas at their site of accumulation, we can cut disease off at the root.

Every day, we have the opportunity to see how the doshas are balanced, according to how we eat, what we eat, and how we are digesting our choices (at both a physical and sensory impression level). We can witness the digestive process by paying attention to our appetite, digestion and elimination. The other pillars of life—sleep and creativity—depend on healthy metabolism so this is an area that deserves our primary attention.

CHAPTER SUMMARY

The gunas and doshas form us and are always at play in our lives. We are born with a unique constitution of metabolic patterns (Prakruti), and these create in us certain tendencies toward specific vulnerabilities. Impacted by the externals and internals of life, the doshas (the biological forces of the elements) move out of their original balance. Ayurveda identifies and treats the imbalanced state (Vikruti), taking into consideration the tendency of the metabolic patterns to reproduce in predictable ways and the three foundational pillars of life: food, sleep and relationship. Through observation and self-awareness, we can begin to identify what is out of balance and why.

SUGGESTED PRACTICE

Start to formally take note of the first two pillars of life—appetite-digestion-elimination and sleep.

Chart the information in a journal: how often you feel hungry during the day and what food you desire, how it satisfies your hunger and for how long. Are you able to have at least one regular daily bowel movement? If not, consider talking with an Ayurveda practitioner for help with nutrition choices and support through herbal medicines.

Also track your levels of energy throughout the day, your ability to get to sleep at night and sleep undisturbed through the night and how you feel upon awakening each morning.

Student Story—Always Learning the Lesson

I had been sober for about six years when I took a deep dive into Yoga, after a lifetime of just splashing around in it. A close call with ovarian cancer inspired the dive. Cancer got my attention the way alcoholism had. When I recovered from cancer, I was on the cusp of midlife and determined to always say yes to the things that called my heart. Yoga did that. I continued my career in journalism as I pursued a basic teacher-training course, studied far and wide, subsequently opened three Yoga studios, became a teacher in research studies of Yoga for cancer patients and taught ongoing classes for cancer patients.

I had stayed close to the AA program and began to see remarkable parallels between the principles of AA and the tenets of Yoga.

In the summer of 2007, I took Durga's Yoga of Recovery course. Even though I was abstinent from alcohol, I was addicted to so many things: work, television, coffee. I loved the course and began to teach and use many of the principles right away. But being a Rajasic, Pitta alcoholic, I was still bound for trouble.

Two years later, in the midst of moving my household, I impulsively grabbed a heavy box of books and felt a little zing in my low back. I kept working, angry at my husband for moving too slowly. I was seething and hurting. I woke up the next day with acute sciatica, quickly followed by a prescription for painkillers—and a new taste for drugs. I don't remember the exact teaching, but at the time what rang in my head was Durga saying something like: If we don't treat our pain, physical or psychic, we will use drugs or alcohol again. Somewhere inside, I knew that even after all the years of recovery and Yoga, I didn't really take proper care of myself. I pushed too hard in the physical world. I kept my emotions down, down, down. I didn't ask for what I needed. I acted like I was fine, I could take care of myself.

I spent the subsequent four or five years in denial about my drug dependency. I hid the drug use until my self-loathing overcame me and I got an AA/NA sponsor to help me with that. The last time Durga and I met in person, she kindly pointed out to me that I had many opportunities in my life to do Sattvic practices and that, really, as we age, that's where we need to put our focus.

I think that, though it takes me a while, I always learn the lesson. The past eight years of recovery from opioid addiction have been the best of my life. I am closer to my husband. I am doing the most meaningful work I can imagine and YoR is a vivid and crucial thread in the tapestry of my life.

Lynn F.

ENDNOTE

1   Svoboda, "Ayurveda: An alternative or complementary medicine?"

Chapter 12

ONE DAY AT A TIME

REMEMBER THAT THE EFFECTS OF TIME AND ENVIRONMENT are the third cause of disease according to Ayurveda. In the AA Big Book, we are told that alcoholism (and other addiction) is progressive, meaning that one of the signs that it is the disease of addiction, rather than situational increased use, is that over time, it tends to get worse, not better. Time is a significant factor in the cause of disease and, on the flipside, it can also be a very helpful guidepost for how we introduce better balance and rhythms into our lives.

In YoR, our solution allows us to make use of the healing aspect of time through a shift in perspective—to see time as an ally, not an enemy. We look at the doshas throughout our lifetime, the seasons of the year, the monthly (moon) cycle, and throughout each day. We connect with the rhythm of life that governs the wisdom of the daily routines (Dinacharya) and seasonal routines (Ritucharya) of Ayurveda.

STAGES OF LIFE

In understanding our elemental nature, Ayurveda describes human development through the stages of life, from Kapha to Pitta to Vata, that each person experiences. The scene that Ayurveda and Yoga set around the story of time helped me tremendously. There are many layers and facets to it. From the Ayurveda perspective we go through three stages of life: the growth phase, the maintenance phase and the degenerative phase. The first is childhood where the growth rate is greatest (anabolic), the second stage is from puberty to around 50 where growth is roughly equal to the rate of breakdown (metabolic maintenance) and the third stage is our senior years where the rate of degeneration exceeds the rate of growth (catabolic). These stages of life mirror the effects of the biological forces of the three doshas—Kapha, Pitta and Vata.

The effect of time is a reality of life and a contributing factor in the disease-causing process. Childhood has different illnesses (frequent colds, runny noses, coughs and excess mucus) than senior years (arthritis, joint pain, bone deterioration); midlife we are in the Pitta stage of life—fire which can make us more prone to hyperacidity, heartburn, acid-indigestion, ulcers and inflammation. This knowledge is very useful as we make decisions around our lifestyle choices in the different periods of our life—it's not one way for the whole journey, just like it's not one way for everyone.

Kapha governs the period of our life from conception to adolescence. Kapha dosha is made up of water and earth elements, which make "mud." Kapha governs the substance and structure of the body and its stage of life is governed by growth. It is the only time in our life where it is appropriate for us to gain 120+ pounds in 15–20 years. It is to be hoped that doesn't happen again in any other stage of life!

Transition: There is no precise timing of any of these periods that fits for everyone; we are indicating a general age range. The Kapha stage of life is shifting to the next stage, Pitta, between the ages of 14 to 21 years old. It is perhaps easier to identify for females as menarche (the onset of menstruation), which indicates that the female is moving into the Pitta stage of life.

Adolescence is a difficult time for many of us, a time of great hormonal flux. We are not quite children but also not yet fully arrived into our adulthood. There is a significant incidence of the onset of addiction during these years. Care and guidance are required during this transition. In older cultures, there were rites of passage that took place around this transition point. Many rehabs try to reenact this more traditional wisdom with activities like vision quests and wilderness rehabs. These are avenues to help adolescents and young adults connect more deeply to the natural order of life.

Ayurveda views these transition periods as having an inherent quality of instability (Rajas). Coming of age rituals mark, honor and respect the rites of passage. All rituals indicate an honoring and celebration of stepping over a line into a new way of being. Our tribal ancestors welcomed the budding young adult into the next stage of life by the people already established within that stage of life. It is good to set some honoring of this beyond modern culture's emphasis on the attainment of certain ages that allow us to participate legally in certain activities, like voting, fighting for our country, smoking cigarettes, drinking alcohol and sexual activity.

Pitta governs the middle years. For females, it is often indicated as the period from menarche to menopause. Fire energy is dominant in this time of life. Fire governs transformation and productivity. Here we transform all the nurturing and growth we receive in our early years into caring for our own further education, career, families, children, elders. We can view the Pitta stage of life as the years where we have the capacity for reproduction and creating a life for ourselves. It is a time where the onus rests on us to perform our duty, and care for our own children, as well as our parents and wider community: elders, spiritual teachers and those less able or less financially fortunate than ourselves. This is a time of life marked by giving and charity. It is also a time when we may become imbalanced in Pitta types of diseases like workaholism, chronic inflammation, ulcers and heart attacks.

Transition: Once you are in a phase of life, there is a certain amount of continuity. Transition stages are more problematic. Another transition stage is menopause or man-opause, a time of letting go of our former identities, careers, family status. This can be very challenging for many, especially parents as they face the "empty nest." Sometimes, women are better prepared to embrace a change in pace and focus which may be related to the definite physical experience of the end of the menstrual cycle. I like the book by Joan Borysenko titled *A Woman's Book of Life*, which describes how women grow and change in seven-year cycles throughout their lifespan. Joan describes this period as the birth of the "Guardian."[1] In this "saging" period many women step into their power with more authenticity, integrity and wholeness. They develop a passionate protectiveness, and a capacity to mother the larger world—emanating the energy of the divine feminine, goddess, activist, challenger.

We can cultivate the capacity to embrace our saging years rather than vainly attempting to reclaim our youth through various means (Viagra, cosmetic surgery, a new, younger romantic partner etc.). This time of our life is known in Ayurveda as the Forest Dweller stage (Vanaprastha). For those of us who have children it is said that we enter this stage of life when we see the face of the child of our child, meaning our grandchild's face.

Hopefully now we do not need to exert so much effort in being the breadwinners; we have raised our family and the next generation now assumes those responsibilities. We can rest a little, enjoy the fruits of our labor and turn to our spiritual practices. This is often referred to as "empty nest" time when our children have grown up and left home for college, starting their own career, marriage and family. Many of us find ourselves being drawn to more creative pastimes that we did not have so much time for in our earlier years. Of course, for many experiencing the effects of addiction on the family this may not be the case. Grandparents may be parenting children because the parents are living on the streets, or in hospitals, jails or institutions—the Tamasic destination points that come from the destructive nature of the disease of addiction. This means that these carers need to do their best to bring the life science wisdom and simplicity to themselves and the rest of the family. They especially need to take a few moments for self-care and not run on empty. As we begin to understand the intergenerational nature of the disease of addiction and reduce stigma and discrimination around it we can move toward more help being available for the actual effects on the whole family with more recovery-oriented systems of care (ROSC) and recovery support services (RSS). Here is a short description of these hoped for advances in the field of addiction care:

> A ROSC supports the premise that there are many pathways to recovery. Recovery-oriented activities include providing a menu of traditional treatment services and alternative therapies, including peer recovery coaching, acupuncture, meditation, and music and art therapy. Recovery support services, including employment assistance, child care, care management and housing support, may enhance the engagement of individuals and their families in achieving and sustaining recovery.[2]

For females the **Vata** stage of life governs the period post-menopause; for males it can be thought of as somewhere between 50 to 60 years old. It is the catabolic stage when the breakdown of the body's tissues outweighs the capacity for growth and repair. It is a time to detach from the concerns of raising a family and building a career. Ideally, we can be more generous in our allocation of time for rest, self-care and self-reflection. The last stage in the cycle of life takes us toward death, which according to the Vedas is a dropping of this particular physical body and reincarnating in another suitable form when necessary to proceed on with our soul's evolutionary journey.

In our modern culture youngsters tend to be hurtling themselves at high speed into adulthood, and most of us fear moving out of the productive/ Pitta years. The Vata time of life is of equal importance to the previous stages.

In YoR, rather than using the word aging, we like to call it saging. As our worldly responsibilities decrease, we have more time and energy to transform our lived experience into wisdom to share with younger members of our family and communities. When we live by the belief that spirit is our essential nature we are more able to utilize this time in our lives to foster a more subtle growth—a deeper understanding, generous sharing and loving detachment from our worldly possessions. Think of the Potlatch Ceremony practiced by Indigenous peoples of the Pacific Northwest Coast, a gift-giving feast of giving away treasured possessions to family and friends. This is a great time to release encumbrances that block our forward movement in personal growth.

Ayurveda's view of the stages of life:

▸ Kapha: The growth years.

▸ Pitta: The (re)productive years.

▸ Vata: The saging years.

SEASONS

We move through our lives and mark our recovery milestones year by year. Within each 12-month period we move through different seasons. Ayurveda seasonal routines mostly indicate what types of food to favor according to what is local and in season, and also opportunities to pause from activities at the junction of the seasons to carry out a short cleanse/detoxification.

The term "Ritucharya" means "to be guided by the season." In the West, we can correlate the seasons to the three doshas as follows:

▸ Kapha is late winter/early spring, a time of dormancy, when the moist, cold qualities of Kapha dominate.

▸ Pitta is late spring/summer—warmer weather reflecting the hot quality of Pitta.

▸ Vata is fall/early winter—a season where we are witness to more of the cold, light, dry and mobile qualities of Vata as the leaves fall from the trees and the grasses and plants crunch under our feet.

Variety through Seasonal Food Choices

Very few of us want to hear we can never eat a particular food again but that is often what various diets advise. Ayurveda mitigates this "absolute" rule by taking into account the season in which the food is consumed. Here is a quick glance at this idea:

Kapha—late winter/early spring (approximately March through June). Choose lighter foods toward spring months: berries, grapefruit, lemons, limes, sprouts, greens (collard, kale, dandelions, mustard, spinach, Swiss chard, lettuce, parsley, watercress), asparagus, radishes, turnips. Less wheat.

Pitta—late spring/summer (approximately July through October). Favor cherries, berries, melons, plums, pineapples, broccoli, cauliflower, celery, cilantro, cucumbers, fennel, jicama, zucchini. Less spicy, salty, sour, nuts and fermented products.

Vata—fall/early winter (approximately November through February). Opt for figs, dates, cooked apples, bananas, mangoes, oranges/tangerines, persimmons, beets, avocados, carrots, sweet potatoes, winter squash, pumpkins. Less dry, light, raw foods.

It is beyond the scope of this book to go into great detail about seasonal food choices. Dr. John Douillard's book titled *The 3-Season Diet* is a great resource to help us align our dietary choices to what is happening with the seasons. Seasonal food choice is balancing for us personally and more sustainable for the planet as a whole which is very helpful as we become aware of how adversely affected many areas are becoming by climate change.

As each season is governed by one of the doshas, this offers a way to balance all three doshas over the span of a year. This is most appropriate if we are fairly balanced in our constitution. If we are experiencing doshic imbalance then we are advised to narrow our nutrition choices to foods that balance the particular dosha(s) that is causing our symptomatic concerns. If you are unsure of your dosha, a seasonal approach to our food choices provides a good option as we are never limited to one list of appropriate food; we cycle our choices according to seasonal foods and they often will help us feel more balanced and in tune with the greater cycles of the sun's energy.

Ebb and Flow, Cleanse and Celebrate

Ayurveda views the transition time between seasons as a good time to take a pause to rest and reassess our level of balance, routines and energy levels.

There is a certain continuity when in a season; the potential for imbalance increases as we transition from one season to another. Ideal markers are the fall and spring equinoxes, both good times to do a short cleanse (up to four weeks before/after). A seasonal cleanse is where we follow a mono-diet of kitchari (basmati rice and split mung beans cooked with ghee and spices—see www.yogaofrecovery.com for recipe), for three, five or seven days. Eliminating the wide variety of other food we normally partake in offers rest and repair to the digestive system. Spices and herbs help spark the digestive fire and gently remove toxins through the feces, urine and sweat.

Ayurveda gives us tools to navigate these periods more smoothly. For instance, in spring we can support the body by releasing some of the insulation we have taken on over the winter months, lightening up for summer. Pitta in late spring and early summer melts away the storage of the Kapha—this often results in spring allergies and colds. A short fall cleanse allows us to release excess heat built up over the summer months—it can also be likened to winterizing our home in preparation for the upcoming cold season. Visit www.yogaofrecovery.com for more detailed information on how to do these seasonal cleanses.

Celebrating

It is good to mark our calendars with dates of special remembrance and celebration. The summer and winter solstices are opportunities for celebration. We can shift our choices by noting the marker points of the spring and fall equinox and winter and summer solstice. These can be our indicators throughout the year to honor both full participation and celebration with a few days of withdrawal for cleansing and rebalancing energy in our system. Incorporating this aspect of the dynamic flow of time is a big part of helping us remember that we can get through challenging times and set time aside to recognize and celebrate times that are meaningful to our own personal belief systems, in our own personal way, rather than blindly following the mainstream holidays which may have become triggering and jaded for many of us through the emphasis on over-indulgence and rampant consumerism.

SAD—Seasonal Affective Disorder

This comes up mostly at the transition from the warmer season (Pitta) moving to the prolonged colder seasons of Vata, which includes the holidays, followed by another cold season governed by Kapha. In recovery groups, many people have challenges and there seems to be more relapse as we shift toward the fall/winter season and the holidays. People who live in the colder northern areas often migrate south during the winter season, for instance elderly New Yorkers going to Florida. The ability to opt to go somewhere warmer is a therapy in its own right, but not one available to all of us.

Our emphasis on time encourages us to give attention and prioritize our own special days—what is meaningful for us? Especially in a season we find challenging, it is important to celebrate even our small successes and honor milestone markers of our recovery journey.

Monthly Menstrual (Lunar) Cycle

For women, another cycle that deserves particular attention as we seek a more emotional balance in recovery is the feminine monthly cycle, which relates directly to the lunar cycle. Recovery can feel challenging at certain times in a woman's monthly cycle. Kapha governs the first half of the cycle as the endometrium lining thickens. When ovulation occurs, Pitta dominates—the potential for life exists. If the egg remains unfertilized, the last portion of the cycle is governed by Vata which regulates the flow of menstrual blood.

When we are under stress, we produce stress hormones that block up the biochemical pathways that help with the production of sex hormones. If corticosterone levels rise, reproduction drops. Many females in recovery experience dysregulated menstrual cycles due to the metabolic and hormonal disrepair left behind by overuse/misuse of substances, disordered eating and inadequate self-care as we overwork and overextend our energies to the care of others.

Women often suffer from PMS, or an even more serious condition, PMDD (premenstrual dysphoric disorder). The reason to pay attention to where we are in our monthly cycle is that the symptoms of PMDD mirror those of PAWS (post-acute withdrawal syndrome), the symptoms that occur in early detox and recovery. Adopting a Sattvic lifestyle contributes a great deal to balancing a woman's metabolic and hormonal systems.

I recommend you take the time to read and follow the recommendations offered by Claudia Welch in her excellent book *Balance Your Hormones, Balance Your Life.*

AYURVEDA DETOXIFICATION, PANCHAKARMA

A deep cleanse may be necessary to lighten up our physical state. The process of Panchakarma is a deep detoxification carried out by trained Ayurveda doctors, practitioners and therapists. It is advised for conditions of Ama (toxins) and on a preventive aspect it can be undertaken every two to five years depending on our health history. It is a big undertaking, a deep house cleaning that reverses disease from the roots.

YoR offers an annual detoxification retreat at a rural Ayurveda center in India (Vaidyagrama)[3] where we undertake three to four weeks of physical detoxification and rejuvenation that rebalances the metabolic and hormonal system. Some come to take treatment in an attempt to reduce body pain and avoid limb-replacement surgery. I myself managed to end my reliance on the asthma medication I had been using for most of my life. It is a long overdue aspect of ongoing care for people in recovery to receive all-round holistic health care in a retreat-like setting with a group of people in recovery. We call it our DREAM team: Diet, Rest, Environment and Ayurvedic Medicine. People who undergo treatment are dealing with a variety of concerns—quitting smoking (including cigarettes, vaping and cannabis), coming off an already medically supervised tapered-down dose of Suboxone after a few years of being drug free, coming off various pharmaceuticals (antidepressant/anxiety, sleep, ADHD medicines etc.).

ONE DAY AT A TIME

Time as an ally in our healing and growth process culminates in being able to bring rhythm to our lives "One Day at a Time." We become able to tune into the ability to swim downstream as we become familiar with the flow of the doshas throughout each 24-hour period. This relates to the daily routines and shows their deep impact in addressing all three causes of disease: misuse of the senses, crimes against wisdom and the effects of time and environment.

Dinacharya

Each dosha governs a four-hour period during the day:

▸ Kapha: 6–10 am and 6–10 pm.

▸ Pitta: 10 am–2 pm and 10 pm–2 am.

▸ Vata: 2–6 pm and 2–6 am.

Each particular dosha is dominant for four hours, twice a day. While we have our own innate rhythms, the planetary rhythms are more powerful. Ayurveda asks that we follow nature's rhythms. Artificial rhythms lead to more Rajas in the mind. The first step toward balance is to create a daily routine, a Dinacharya.

We've all had days when we feel our life is still unmanageable when we are unsettled by a sleepless night, afternoon fatigue or nighttime hunger. Rather than this causing a cascade of bad decisions, we look at the clock, ascertain the dosha time of day and pacify in a healthy way knowing this period will last only four hours. This also helps us set our waking and sleep hours to support us so we are not "swimming against the tide."

TYPICAL (UNHEALTHY) MODERN LIFESTYLE

This is a very common lifestyle for millions of people. First, we get up during Kapha time—after 6 am. This means we are having to immediately counter the heavy, stable qualities in the environment; hence, many of us immediately reach for coffee first thing in the morning. Maybe we skip breakfast and eat a cold lunch on the run or at our desk/computer.

By afternoon, between 2 and 4 pm in the Vata time of day, we feel fatigued and grab readily available stimulants to boost our energy (i.e. coffee or sugar or both). Crash-and-crave is often a good description of how we feel during the Vata time of day (2–6 pm). Dr. John Douillard, in his book *The 3-Season Diet*, describes it as reaching for the four Cs during that period: caffeine, candy, cola and chips. In active addiction, there are many more!—cocktails, Chardonnay, cannabis, cocaine/crack etc.

Twelve hours later, many of us also experience sleep difficulties between 2 and 4 am—during the Vata time of night. Observe that Vata has us awake when we want to be sleeping, and drowsy and longing for sleep in the middle of the afternoon. This is an indication of the need to make changes to balance Vata.

In the evening, we eat the largest meal of the day, during Kapha time (6–10 pm) when our digestive power is less strong. We then push past the tiredness that emerges in the Kapha evening hours. Most of us campaigned throughout our childhood years to be allowed to stay up late and we are darn well going to continue with that now we are adults in charge of our schedules!

Perhaps around 9–10 pm we start to get that second wind (just as the Pitta energy is rising) which may keep us up until midnight to 1 am or even 2 am. We may start working on a project, watching TV, Netflix binging, doom scrolling, surfing the internet (porn, conspiracy theories, impulse shopping, cyber stalking, casual hook up on geo-dating sites etc.). This is unwise as Pitta governs the eyes and sense of sight. So many of us have disturbed sleep: we are unable to get to sleep (Pitta) or unable to remain soundly asleep throughout the entire night (Vata). Then this unhealthy cycle starts again the next day.

We can also experience "nighttime eating syndrome" which means that the energy that should be used to cleanse the body overnight is expended on digesting food. The food that we are eating at this time is often not our healthiest choice. Tamas governs the nighttime so we naturally have less capacity to make Sattvic choices after dark—is it just a coincidence that this is the busiest time of the night for ERs and law enforcement? Remember that Tamas Pitta was about violence and destructiveness. My grandmother had a saying that an hour of sleep before midnight was worth two after midnight. Ayurveda's view of time helped me connect with the wisdom she was speaking of—thanks Jeanie!

In recovery, we can attune our lifestyles to supportive routines. Remember that sleep is one of the three pillars. We can remind ourselves with humor to flow with the greater planetary rhythms with the phrase, "Nothing good happens after 10 pm!" Most of us can attest to the fact that what we can easily become engaged in at that time of night is far less attractive or appealing upon arising in the early morning, so best to just go to bed before we trash all our day's efforts by sliding into lesser choices so easily supported in the Tamas time of night.

LETTING YOUR BODY REST

When we sleep, our liver (governed by Pitta dosha) filters through and metabolizes our day's intake. I like the way Jennifer Workman describes this in her book *Stop Your Cravings*:

your liver can perform its cleansing without also having to digest a heavy evening meal at the same time, which would undermine the efficiency of both functions. Have you ever stayed so late in your office that the cleaners couldn't get in to do their job? If so, you certainly noticed that when you arrived the next morning, the trashcan was still overflowing and yesterday's garbage had not been removed. That's exactly what can happen to our bodies if we don't give our liver enough time to "empty the trash" during the night: it's still there when we get up the next morning, so that our stomach might be a bit bloated or our eyes red and puffy.[4]

ESTABLISHING BETTER RHYTHMS RESULTS IN BETTER DAYS

We live in a Rajasic society where everything is full-on 24/7. At first, when we make changes to our daily routines and tend toward our self-care, it may feel self-indulgent—it is not. These Ayurveda routines are deeply therapeutic and healing, promoting healthy growth and mind-body balance. They are intended to bring us closer to the natural rhythms of the universe, of which we are an organic part.

A HEALTHY DAILY SCHEDULE

▸ Get up during Vata time, before 6 am. The earlier we rise, the more precious time we have for our daily routines of self-care and meditation first thing in the morning.

▸ Undertake our most vigorous physical exercise or physical work during the 6–10 am Kapha time. Eat a light breakfast.

▸ Pitta relates to metabolizing mental experiences, so do our most arduous mental work during Pitta time and also eat our largest meal of the day at lunchtime when the digestive fire is strong.

▸ In the Vata time of day (2–6 pm), honor the fact we may feel a dip in energy. Dr. John Douillard indicates that the brain uses 80 percent of the body's glycogen, or energy supplies, during this time.[5] If it doesn't get it, cravings arise.

　－ Vata is light and creative, so it is not time to tackle our tax return. This is where distraction, time-wasting and procrastination start to plague our feeling of self-efficacy. Better to have tackled mentally demanding work in the Pitta time of day and not leave it until late afternoon to face.

- Vata time can be good for creative planning or even routine tasks. Take a Vata-pacifying snack; consider Yoga Nidra, a walk in nature or an Abhyanga (self-massage) at this time. Since Vata is cold, light, dry and mobile, choosing these activities reduces Vata. Stay away from stimulants and offer our system some short rest and deep nurturing practices.

▸ Have a light supper in the earlier Kapha evening hours. If absolutely necessary, we can exercise during this time but morning is preferable. Allow three hours between supper and bedtime; this allows us to digest the day's activities during the Pitta (liver) time of night (10 pm–2 am).

▸ Aim to get to bed during Kapha time (before 10 pm). We can save ourselves a lot of effort or great feats of willpower by sleeping at this time.

▸ Ayurveda recommends getting up before 6 am. If we have gone to bed before 10 pm, we will have had eight hours of sleep. If we get up in Vata time (before 6 am), we assist one of the major functions of the Vata dosha, the elimination of waste products, urine and feces. Simply arising earlier can cure long-standing constipation problems.

COUNTER AND CAPITALIZE ON THE DOSHA ENERGY

Kapha

If we have excess Kapha, it is important to engage in activities that counter Kapha during the Kapha times of day; for instance, it may be possible to lose weight purely by shifting the time of meals, eating only between the hours of 10 am and 6 pm. In the evening, we can capitalize on Kapha by going to bed when we feel the waves of tiredness, even if it is as early as 8–10 pm. Kapha is the dosha that best supports sleep. Before bed, gentle activities like restorative exercise, Yoga and meditation are all good.

Pitta

If we have excess Pitta, it is important to engage in activities that reduce Pitta as we approach the Pitta time of evening. Counter the fire energy by turning off all media screens at least one hour before bed. Aim to be in bed by 9.30 pm and sleeping by 10 pm.

In the daytime, we can capitalize on Pitta by eating our largest meal or performing our most mentally demanding work.

Vata

Many of us have a Vata imbalance, so continuous Vata-balancing activities are important. Counter Vata in the afternoon by lessening the demands we make on ourselves during these hours and set up a more easeful transition time from work to rest. A light Vata-pacifying drink like warmed (almond) milk with spices is a good way to nourish rather than stimulate. This is also a good time for Yoga Nidra. At work, catching up on filing or doing other activities that do not expend a lot of mental energy may be helpful.

As we gradually find a more healthy rhythm in our lives one of the greatest rewards for many is that we are able to restore ourselves fully by sleeping through the night allowing us to awaken refreshed with energy to face the radiance of a new day before 6 am.

TYING IT ALL TOGETHER

As we bring more Ayurveda into our life and work to cumulatively balance the doshas in our mind-body system, we'll become aware of which seasons, times of day, times of month create the most imbalance for us. Pay attention to the times when we experience symptoms of imbalance, detecting the symptoms through the felt sensations of qualities (cold/hot, mobile/stable, heavy/light etc.)—this will help us ascertain the dosha(s) that has gone out of balance. Next, address the imbalance by applying the rule of opposites to reduce/pacify, especially during the peak time of that dosha in the 24-hour daily cycle.

As we start to become aware, we can tackle any imbalance during our own daily self-care, daily routines, and, as needed, with the guidance of Ayurveda doctors, and perhaps for some of us with a Panchakarma (three to four weeks of actual treatment). There are many levels of care. This is the beauty of

Ayurveda; we don't have to be at death's door to increase our level of care, nor do we have to wait until we have a disease diagnosed. We can begin right now, make a choice today; notice when we start feeling stressed or out of balance and feel into what is needed. Ayurveda is preventative, rejuvenative and therapeutic. It offers a continuum of care perfectly meeting the different needs we experience on our recovery journey.

Time is an important factor both in the disease of addiction and recovery from addiction. The emphasis in recovery on "One Day at a Time" encourages us to pick back up and restart if we lapse (relapse)—one breath, one stretch, one meal, one 6 am wake-up alarm at a time. This is one of the gifts of Ayurveda; it is not so much a black and white, on the wagon off the wagon deal, but more of a continuously available self-empowering choice.

CHAPTER SUMMARY

Addiction and disease are progressive: over time, they get worse. Our modern culture is deeply time-imbalanced, causing us to feel that we do not have enough of it, need to fill it, and move at faster and faster speeds. Ayurveda is rooted in nature and natural rhythms, providing a road map for understanding and working with the stages of life we all pass through (and their elemental and doshic influences). Ayurveda also promotes alignment with nature's rhythms through seasonal routines (Ritucharya) and through important daily self-care routines (Dinacharya) that establish and support health and well-being, creating a deeper, more personal relationship with time.

SUGGESTED PRACTICE

During the Vata time of day, offer your system some short rest and deep nurturing practices. Eat a Vata-pacifying snack; consider Yoga Nidra or a restorative Yoga practice, a walk in nature or an Abhyanga (self-massage) at this time. See www.yogaofrecovery.com for instructions for simple Abhyanga.

Student Story—Remembering Our Innate Wisdom

Being an adult child of an alcoholic, when I came to Yoga of Recovery, I was very familiar with 12-Step programs. I was also an experienced Yoga teacher. Yet I had hit a wall a number of years prior with the discovery of a loved one's addiction. However you say it, addiction is a spiritual malady, or spiritual ignorance, or forgetting that our true nature is spirit, clearly a spiritual process is the solution for recovery. As Durga says, "we have this innate wisdom but we've forgotten."

The daily practices that Ayurveda suggests and YoR teaches help to ground and calm my Vata/Pitta tendencies and restore me to a sense of balance. There is no one silver bullet but the wide range of small, simple practices add up to a whole life change. As a result, I have been able to create a peaceful Sattvic environment in my home and life as a result of this knowledge. I have tools that I can put in place when life throws me a curve ball, whether it's spending some time in nature, buying myself fresh flowers or just taking a deep breath.

YoR helped me renew my relationship with my AA program, deepened my Yoga practice and enhanced my recovery as I put the practices to work. Understanding Yoga philosophy and the way the gunas and doshas relate also help me to infuse the Yoga classes that I teach with greater compassion. The experience of joining Durga for Panchakarma in India was extremely beneficial and made me understand how important it is to create a daily routine for self-care. Through YoR, I now have an international support community for which I am eternally grateful.

Celia B.

Student Story—My True Nature as Spirit

I began my Yoga journey in 2011 after a long career in corporate America. As a codependent, addicted to external love relations, during my life I developed many unhealthy attachments and addictions. Yoga and meditation awakened me to my spiritual roots. In 2019, I began to integrate Ayurveda daily lifestyle practices introduced through Yoga of Recovery studies with Durga. These practices include dietary, physical and spiritual components that are now part of my daily life. They allow me to awaken to my "true nature as spirit" and work to balance the needs of my human life experience and longings of the heart, without unhealthy attachments and addictions. Practicing truth and light every day builds my resilience, helping me to overcome my addictions "one day at a time."

Gary S.

ENDNOTES

1   Borysenko, J. (1998) *A Woman's Book of Life: The Biology, Psychology and Spirituality of the Feminine Life Cycle.* New York: Riverhead Books, p. 153.
2   SAMHSA (2010) *Recovery-Oriented Systems of Care (ROSC) Resource Guide.* www.samhsa. gov/sites/default/files/rosc_resource_guide_book.pdf
3   http://vaidyagrama.com
4   Workman, J. (2001) *Stop Your Cravings: The Ayurvedic Plan for Losing Body Fat, Increasing Energy, and Using Food to Manage Stress.* New York: Free Press, p. 12.
5   Douillard, J. (2001) *The 3 Season Diet: Eat the Way Nature Intended: Lose Weight, Beat Food Cravings, and Get Fit.* New York: Random House, p. 158.

Chapter 13

DIGESTION UNDER STRESS

W E ARE DEVELOPING DAILY ROUTINES and beginning to experience and notice changes and there is always something that disrupts our new efforts—a trip, a person, a deadline. These added demands can easily get us off track. We can bring an Ayurvedic perspective to their impact, especially on the digestive system, and learn how to recognize symptoms and imbalances early on.

AYURVEDA AND DIGESTION

Ayurveda nutrition therapy starts with digestion. Ayurveda supports the creation of health by focusing on metabolism, and one of the foundational metabolic systems is digestion. Therefore, bringing awareness to our digestion is critical.

In Chapter 11, we saw that food is the first of Ayurveda's pillars of life (along with sleep and relational health/proper energy management around all our relationships). You may recall that each dosha is associated with a primary site located along the digestive tract. By paying attention to these sites and the dosha accumulating there, we can begin to take remedial action more promptly. The first signs of imbalance are: Vata manifesting as gas in the large intestine, Pitta as hyperacidity from excess bile and acids from the small intestine, and Kapha as phlegm and mucus in the stomach and chest area. Treating the doshas at this early stage enables us to stop the progression of disease.

AMA

Ama is a Sanskrit word that refers to the toxic residue left behind when food is improperly digested. Ama is like a pathogen; it breeds toxins and disturbs immunity. It overflows from the digestive system and coats the cells, enters the tissues and channels and interferes with the body's normal functioning. This is why it is so important to catch the first disturbances within the digestive system.

The main signs of ama include:

▸ coated tongue (this is why tongue scraping is so useful)

▸ foul smelling feces, urine, sweat

▸ bad breath that is not related to food or tooth decay

▸ body odor that is not eliminated by bathing.

Some secondary signs and symptoms:

▸ fatigue

▸ feeling blocked/congested

▸ feeling groggy on waking

▸ frequent digestive symptoms

▸ frequent excess salivation

▸ weakened immune system.

If you can't digest the food you are eating—no matter how "good" you think the food is, or the nutritional "experts" have told you the food is—it is not good for you. When we have symptoms and eat the foods anyway, we are disengaging our intellect from our actions, a clear example of "crimes against wisdom."

AGNI—DIGESTIVE FIRE

We often hear "you are what you eat;" Ayurveda says, "you are what you digest." Agni is the Sanskrit word used to indicate overall digestive fire. It means the "transforming will or force" and is a primary determinant of good health. Agni enables us to absorb nutrients properly and overcome many of the pathogens that may be in our food.

In making our nutritional choices, it helps to bring attention to this power of transformation available to us through the foods we eat. Rather than feeding our outwardly focused mind with all of the Rajasic and Tamasic "food" options offered by modern culture, we can feed our bodies Sattvic food and create more clarity of mind and emotions, and even nourish our inner spiritual aspirations.

The qualities of agni are hot, light, sharp, dry and penetrating. We pose a challenge to our ability to digest when we take in foods and beverages with the opposite qualities to agni, such as cold and/or heavy food, iced beverages.

We find the qualities of agni in abundance in spices; hence, we make use of spices to enhance our ability to digest food. One of the most considerable practicalities of Ayurveda is that our first medicine cabinet is our kitchen, not only the food but how we spice our meals.

We generally lose our appetite when feeling unwell—this is because it is the fire energy that tackles the virus or pathogen, so there is little fire left for digestion. There is a direct correlation between agni and immunity. If we consume foods that are hard to digest, over time it is likely we'll compromise our immunity. When we are ill, light foods, warm drinks and pungent spices such as ginger, turmeric, black pepper, cardamom and cinnamon are helpful.

THE STATES OF AGNI AND HELPFUL SPICES

Agni has four states: balanced, variable, high and low.

When our **agni is balanced**, we are blessed with regular appetite; we experience physical hunger and have a desire for food two to three times a day. We have regular bowel movements (at least one per day) and no bloating or gas. Our mind is sharp and clear. To maintain balanced agni, we can use mild Sattvic spices such as fennel, cumin, coriander, turmeric, cardamom. A simple agni-supportive tea can be made by adding one teaspoon each of the seeds of cumin, coriander and fennel in four to six cups of water in a pot on the stove top, bring to a boil and allow five to ten minutes to infuse.

Variable agni is most prominent in Vata types, but not exclusively as the Vata dosha is mobile and is prone to imbalance in all types. With variable agni, we experience swings in appetite—ranging from no appetite to suddenly feeling ravenous. It can manifest in gas, constipation, variable circulation, variability in disease resistance and long-term disturbance of the nervous system. Helpful spices include: asafoetida/hing, ginger, cumin, rock salt—all spices that are not overly hot. Hingvastak, an Ayurveda digestive formula, is helpful. It is best to buy digestive formulas as powders and take a little in a half cup of hot water with meals to aid digestion (please visit www.yogaofrecovery.com to link to online retailers such as Banyan Botanicals for all the spice formulas mentioned in this chapter).

The qualities of agni resemble the qualities of Pitta dosha; hence, **high agni** is common in Pitta types. It manifests as excessive appetite, loose stools, maybe diarrhea or heartburn. With this type of digestive fire, it is best to avoid most spices, although a few spices like cumin, coriander and fennel can be used to enhance the flavor of food. Avipattikar is a formula that can be used to remove excess heat from the GI tract and promotes normal, comfortable levels of acidity in the stomach and intestines.

Low agni manifests in poor appetite and is common in Kapha types. Symptoms include low metabolism, tendency toward weight gain, excess mucus and congestion. All spices are generally good. I recommend the classical digestive formula called Trikatu, "the three pungents," long pepper (pippali), ginger and black pepper.

A good first response to any sign of imbalance in our ability to digest our food is simply to make use of spices or a small amount of Ayurveda digestive formulas to remedy the upset. We also need to consider what we are eating and whether a particular food is suitable for our current state of balance. Of course, it is also a very good idea to work with an Ayurveda practitioner or doctor to be guided on the use of spices and our food choices.

HYPOGLYCEMIA

There is a high incidence of hypoglycemia in people recovering from alcohol or substance use disorders as well as eating disorders. In simple terms hypoglycemia is the body's inability to properly handle the large amounts of sugar that the average person consumes today. It's brought on and exacerbated by an overload of sugar, caffeine, tobacco, alcohol and stress. The brain depends on sugar (glucose) almost exclusively; it can't make its own glucose and is 100%

dependent on the rest of the body for its supply. If for some reason the glucose level in the blood falls (or if the brain's requirements increase and demands are not met), there can be effects on the function of the brain.

Some of the symptoms of hypoglycemia include fatigue, mood swings, headaches, sudden hunger, a craving for sweets, irritability or inner trembling. The first thing to do is work towards reducing and eliminating the substances that aggravate this imbalance most: sugar, white flour, caffeine, alcohol and tobacco. It is best to also avoid dried fruits and eat only a small amount of fresh fruit. Again, we tend to think of these as "good" foods but that is not so when hypoglycemia is suspected. Around 95% of alcoholics are hypoglycemic and it's unclear if this was the case before they started drinking, a reason why alcohol became so attractive, or if it resulted from drinking (or using drugs).

According to Ayurveda, hypoglycemia is common in people with a Pitta constitution or a Pitta imbalance, often associated with high agni. Increased Pitta stimulates the secretion of insulin, which lowers the blood sugar level and creates hypoglycemia, which then induces the secretion of adrenaline, which causes rapid heartbeat and tremors. If you are experiencing the symptoms of hypoglycemia, Pitta-pacifying choices in diet with proper scheduling of meals can help to address the imbalance. Stay away from hot spicy foods, fermented food, sour and citrus fruits, and alcohol, smoking cigarettes, sugar and coffee. Drink licorice tea (using one level teaspoon of cut and sifted licorice root per cup of water). This tea will safely increase your blood sugar level. However, individuals with high blood pressure/hypertension should use licorice tea only sparingly; it increases water retention and may raise blood pressure.

DIGESTION UNDER STRESS

We live our lives in forgetfulness of our true nature; hence, we live in the illusion of separation, and thus our automatic, subconscious instinctual drive is focused on survival. We share this level of operation with animals; there is a part of our nature that lives by the law of "eat or be eaten." When our sense of self is dependent on the maintenance of externals, risk of loss is inherent and therefore fear is a persistent background, leading to stress.

The work of Nobel-Prize winner in Physiology or Medicine Hans Selye, and before that of Walter Cannon, introduced the concept of stress into our view of disease. Selye borrowed the term stress from engineering; it originally related to structures like bridges and their ability to bear the load. Stress therefore refers to the body's ability to adapt to the demands put on it—it was named the general adaptation syndrome.

There are two kinds of stress: eu-stress and dis-stress. Eustress is a term for positive/beneficial stress which is defined as moderate psychological stress that is short term and within our coping abilities. In these situations, we adapt; feeling motivated, focusing energy, with the challenge leading to some kind of achievement or improvement. Examples would be undertaking an educational qualification, taking a new job, receiving a promotion at work, learning a new hobby and also marriage, buying a home, having a child, retiring etc.

Distress, however, indicates negative stress when we are unable to adapt as the challenge is outside of our coping abilities; it feels unpleasant, causes anxiety and actually decreases our performance and leads to mental and physical problems. This can be short or long term. Examples would be legal problems, unemployment, debt/bankruptcy/money problems and also filing for divorce, illness, injury or loss of loved one, conflict in relationships and sleep problems etc.—many of these are side-effects of the disease of addiction.

Stressors are not always external; they can be internal. Rajasic feelings and thoughts may include unrealistic expectations, perfectionism and worry as well as habitual behaviors, like enabling, people-pleasing, procrastination and poor boundaries.

We have discussed adaptation and response from the perspective of the gunas, Sattva being the source of spontaneous and adequate response. In Rajas, the mind is like a pendulum swinging between likes and dislikes, highs and lows and the physiology struggles; there is a stress reaction, a failure to adapt, and this leads to patterns of imbalance.

Change is universal and the way we adapt differs from person to person. Many of our adaptive patterns are innate properties of our doshic constitution, biological instinctual drives, and some are learned behaviors, as we have to adapt and cooperate with other people and various circumstances.

THE DOSHAS, DIGESTION AND STRESS

When an organism fails to adapt to its changing environment, whether external changes or internal changes, disease-causing patterns result. For instance, as we transition from one season to another there is a need to adapt to the external environment and make appropriate changes. This is why Ayurveda favors seasonal food choices and cleanses at the junction of the seasons.

The Gut Is Known as the "Second Brain"

We saw in Chapter 5 that a large number of brain receptor sites are associated with the sense and motor organs, particularly the mouth, eyes and hands. Hence, our daily routines are daily brain care. We are now adding the understanding that our nervous system also operates in the gut, where the three doshas have their primary site of accumulation. We also know that stress immediately impacts the digestive system. What does this mean? The doshas are metabolic patterns, each composed of two elements, therefore having recognizable qualities and somewhat predictable tendencies in both physical and psychological response. The tendencies of the doshas under stress are:

▶ Vata: Anxious and/or worried. Tends to have a variable appetite and tends to be chronically activated in "fright-flight" mode.

▶ Pitta: Irritable and/or aggressive. Tends to have a strong/high appetite and tends to be chronically activated in "fight" mode.

▶ Kapha: Needs to pause, tends to get quiet, mull it over. Tends to have a low but constant appetite and tends to be chronically activated in "tend and befriend" mode.

Stuck in Tamas

Most people assign "freeze" to Kapha but it is best not to overlook that Kapha also has a Rajas/overactivation state just like the other two doshas. Freeze/fold is mostly the level of Tamas, and it affects all three doshas. It is when we see a more rigid self-identity or exhaustion of the physiological system. Tamas is the downregulated state when the system is depleted of energy. Freeze often means the inappropriate stress response becomes locked into place as a negative bio-feedback loop: Vata with erratic impulsive behavior, seeking escape; Pitta determined to "win" at any price, compulsive, competitive and intense; Kapha's emotional attachments and possessions now smothering them and those around them.

A coping mechanism dominated by Tamas is freeze/feigning death. We remain locked into our inappropriate stress reactions, now with more of a more despairing and desolate attitude. We may be waiting for others or the world to change to release us rather than actively engaging, acting through our own agency and courage to change. In all cases, we need to remember that our "stuckness" (Tamas) is mental and the change that is most needed is a new attitude/perspective that leads to action.

Tamas is described as the energy that holds improper choices in place. Clients often tell me up front that they refuse to give up certain things that they like to eat and drink. What's interesting to me is that they are often campaigning for the very items that are creating or strongly contributing to the imbalance they seek to resolve. This has led me to query: "What prompts this organism to fight for the right to damage/destroy itself?" I can only surmise that it's the stress talking! A dosha, rather than our discriminating intellect, is driving the bus!

▶ When Vata "drives the bus" they believe they do better with food that is cold, light, dry and often skip meals or eat on the run. They tend to under-eat as they prioritize multi-tasking, keeping busy, expending energy in movement and activity.

▶ When Pitta "drives the bus," they choose spicy, greasy, acidic foods; they are driven, ambitious, goal-oriented, competitive.

▶ When Kapha "drives the bus," they tend toward heavy, comfort foods, sweet foods, baked goods, eating too much and/or too regularly, especially for their sedentary lifestyle.

This is why it is important to bring some remembrance, reverence and respect back to our relationship with food and pay attention to our digestive systems.

Science has shown that stress impairs digestion and the reproductive system; if our sympathetic nervous system is chronically activated, there is reduced energy to digest, rest, or reproduce. Under stress, each dosha manifests differently in how they turn to or turn away from food. In general, Vata tends to under-eat and Pitta and Kapha tend to over-eat; either way, digestive disturbance is the first sure sign that the doshas are starting to imbalance. As a rule of thumb for early detection of imbalance, remember that:

▶ Imbalanced Vata shows up as digestive symptoms such as flatulence/gas, abdominal bloating, pain, belching air.

▸ Imbalanced Pitta shows up as digestive symptoms such as acidity, burning, excess hunger.

▸ Imbalanced Kapha's symptoms are feelings of heaviness, sluggishness, sleepiness, mucus/phlegm and congestion.

FOOD CHOICES OFTEN FUND THE STRESS REACTION

Vata needs to know they can escape, so they choose foods that are light and dry, to support their flight reaction. Pitta is funding the fight reaction, choosing fiery foods, greasy, sour, pungent foods. They are subconsciously feeding their own inflammation, which expands the tissues, and creates more red color which may help to scare others off—similar to the instinctual reaction of many creatures which become red and puffed up when faced with a predator. Perhaps Pitta is choosing their food in the hope that people will feel scared of them and therefore stay away, i.e. "Get too close and I will attack." Kapha's activation is to tend and befriend as they do not have lightness to allow for flight or fierceness that provokes a fight reaction. Kapha tries to smooth things over by presenting a sweetness but it is superficial and fake, not truly heartfelt. They become people pleasers who lose connection to their authentic self as they maintain this mask of self-effacing sweetness which is a fabricated/false self. They tend to reach out for comfort foods with heavy qualities, as they hunker down, waiting for the storm to blow over and things to be safe and comfortable again.

Let's sum up how these imbalances can progress when the food choice is subconsciously funding the stress reaction of the dosha:

▸ Vata types may begin to have a "**fear**" of food. It causes them pain and they feel enormous when their abdomen is bloated, which again makes it more appealing for them to skip food, which aggravates Vata even more. As Vata chooses inappropriate foods, they become increasingly light and dehydrated.

▸ Pittas are known for their strong hunger, intensity and competitiveness and they choose foods that "**fuel**" their fire which leaves them even more heated and hungry. They move into increasing systemic inflammation.

▸ Under stress Kapha is activated but waiting it out, and they see food as perhaps their only true "**friend**." They move into increasing congestion and accumulation.

EATING DISORDERS

As we progress further or engage for longer periods with these inappropriate coping mechanisms around food, our relationship with food can become a diagnosable eating disorder (which is a further progression of the disordered eating that most of us have as a baseline reaction to stress). Vata tends toward anorexia nervosa; this however is not sustainable in the long run, so they may then move to more of a mix of restricting and binging along with bulimic behaviors.

Like Vata, Pitta also has the quality of lightness; they may "aspire" to anorexia, but their strong hunger forces them to eat. As a result, they may binge-eat, then hate themselves for this failure and aim to regain "control" by purging. Kapha tends toward emotional over-eating with weight gain, largely unaware it is a problem.

VANITY AND APPEARANCES

For many people, much of our mental distress is tied up with how we look—which is often primarily gauged by how much we weigh, how our face looks and the condition of our skin. "I feel fat" has become an overall statement made by many of us that incorporates a whole host of emotions. We may actually be feeling any or many of a whole range of uncomfortable emotions: rejected, lazy, angry, disappointed, sad, envious, betrayed, ashamed, unworthy, overwhelmed, less than or guilty. However, we don't know if we are "allowed" to feel this or how to express what we are really feeling so we just attack ourselves with a catch-all comment of self-condemnation from our fat-phobic culture.

Because we are predominantly ego-based, coupled with the media's obsession with physical appearance, we all like to look good—and this can be a bit of a life-saver in relation to how long some of us manage to continue to show up in the world when addictions begin to affect our appearance. Consider "Your Face on Meth," an app developed in 2013.[1] The designers hoped the app would be used in schools to educate teenagers on the dangers of meth use. Users upload a photo and can see in seconds how the drug destroys their looks. They see a dramatic demonstration of the immense physical toll that drugs like meth can have on appearance and thereby get an eyeful of the seriousness of addiction. Eventually, all addictions take a physical toll, not just on how we look but on our key metabolic functions. That's why this Ayurveda perspective is so helpful for us in recovery to reclaim health.

There is a doshic aspect to the vanity most of us have around appearances. It is important to consider this as it relates in many ways to addiction: many of us believe we need to look a certain way in order to be loved and accepted and we have the false perception that if we look okay, then everything is okay.

▸ Vata tends to be thinner with a slight body frame. They feel rewarded by lightness and like to feel free and unfettered. Vata's "look" is often the most independent as they don't place much value on fitting in and may have their own quirky, rebellious sense of style.

▸ Pitta is often vain and likes to be presentable. They tend to emphasize good color-coordination and like to dress and appear properly put together. They appreciate proper function and form from their clothing, and if they find something that works for them—meets whatever exacting standards they have in their mind—they may buy it in a few colors. If they are focused on their goals they may even decide on a specific outfit or look and wear a version of it every day so as not to waste their time or energy in frivolous fashion decisions.

▸ Although Kapha naturally have a larger body size than the other two doshas, they are known to be graceful in movement. Their porcelain skin and lustrous hair are sought after in our standardized idea of beauty. They can carry a considerable amount of weight gain fairly well, choosing clothes that are loose (quite feminine and flowing in the case of female Kaphas, accentuating their bosom and round hips).

RAJAS AND WEIGHT

The progression of the Rajas guna brings vigilance, arousal, activation and mobilization. Biochemically, there is an internal physiological response—paired with the interpretation of what the stress is from an emotional level. How we interpret a situation has a lot to do with our genetics, life history and what has built up as inappropriate stress reactions already within us.

We can begin to pay more attention and notice our cravings and how they change depending on what is stressing us and how extreme the situation is. There are three ways stress can impact our body weight:

▶ Loss of appetite: Generally this is natural when it is a short-term response—the digestive fire is unavailable while the system deals with more immediate demands of the stressor. It becomes problematic when it is chronically activated.

▶ Food cravings: Through the connection of the gunas and doshas we understand cravings to be an acute/sudden activation and motivation (Rajas), toward a substance the imbalanced dosha has fixated on which tends to be mirroring its own qualities—light, dry and crunchy (Vata); hot, spicy, salty, fried (Pitta); and sweet, heavy, comfort food (Kapha). The Rajas effect makes it feel urgent and overrides reason, resolve and will. Over time Tamas sets in to undermine efforts to change, keeping the inappropriate choices locked in place.

▶ Emotional eating. This is a way to find short-term comfort, stuffing down our emotions. We are fixing our emotional needs with a physical response and the availability of food makes this very easy to do, at any time of the day or night.

SHIFTS AND SOLUTIONS

It is important to consider our stress reactions and how they affect our food choices and habits. When we have cravings for certain foods, or experience certain times we want to eat (not from physical hunger), or skip eating altogether, the first thing to do is simply become aware of it without judgment. Just notice the pattern. As we know now what is at the root of these issues/choices—imbalanced agni and doshas in reaction to our faulty perceptual process (Rajas and Tamas)—we can start to take appropriate action to return to balance.

The reason most diets don't work is that we can't get ourselves to follow a diet, even when it makes sense to us on a rational and logical level, until we understand and accept our reactions to perceived stress. Many of us have grown up with the sense that the world is unreliable and unpredictable. There is a complex intertwining of our biology and our emotions and the endless way our feelings and personalities impact our bodies. A neat and tidy one size fits all diet protocol doesn't work because we are not all the same; change is constant.

What we can do is build up our understanding of how all these variables push us toward certain tendencies and see how they play out in our lives, in relation to our food choices, digestion and stress. We can pay attention to where we are on our own journey. This is a unique, dynamic and empowering aspect of Ayurveda.

It is very difficult to attain lasting change with regard to our food choices without stress management and spiritual remembrance. In this dynamic, ever-changing world, we can return to the philosophy of who we are through spiritual practice such as meditation, and employ stress management practices like Yoga Nidra and the Inner Resource Meditation.

BODY SENSATION PRACTICE

It is important to make contact with ourselves to be able to gauge our gut reaction, the visceral feeling within us as we bring different situations into our minds. It helps to ascertain *where* they appear in the body and *how* they appear—what is the actual felt sensation. Here it may be useful to remind yourself of the vocabulary of the 20 qualities/ten pairs of opposites of the five elements (here they are: cold/hot, wet/dry, heavy/light, static/mobile, dense/flowing, gross/subtle, dull/sharp, soft/hard, smooth/rough and cloudy/clear). Feel into it as it appears; if you find a sensation of heat, after you have allowed yourself to feel that sensation, just as it is, meeting it with curiosity, then allow yourself to find its opposite—a sense of coolness somewhere in the body, and again meet and greet that sensation, with the idea that there is no need to fix or change it. This allows us to bring some balance. In between reactivity and repression, there is a balanced place to be—this is our capacity to work with practices to increase Sattva.

You might work with a recent, happy moment, then a recent moment of mild stress or challenge, and when you feel ready, bring to mind a long-standing resentment or misunderstanding and find where it is located in the body and what sensation arises with it. Make a commitment to check in with the body as you become aware of your mind telling you that you're "stressed." This is a practice you can engage in any time, any place. It is important to slow down to be able to sense and notice this intimate connection between our stress reaction and metabolism.

Awareness of Our Food and How We Eat

As we shop for groceries we can become aware of all of the people who have contributed to making it available for us. Of course, the more local and fresh food we can find, the better. As we eat our meals, eat slowly and offer gratitude for the food, and allow time for the food to digest.

Appetite, Digestion and Elimination

It is best to eat fresh foods in their natural state as these tend to be more Sattvic and higher in prana (the vital life force). Choose food that is free of additives, preservatives and pesticides as much as possible. Remember Sattvic food is an offering to us by the planet—to keep us here, embodied.

Pause

It is helpful to have go-tos for those moments when stress threatens to take over and derail us. Here are a number of suggestions for ways to pause and make another choice:

- Take a moment to check into what body sensations are present—where are they located, and what are their qualities?

- Take a moment to sense into our breathing.

- Hydrate—drink a glass of room temperature water.

- Lubricate with healthy oils—both internal and external—apply oil to our hands, feet, body.

- Connect with all five senses:

  - five things you can see

  - four things you can touch

- three things you can hear

- two things you can smell

- one thing you can taste.

▸ Get up and move.

▸ Go outside into nature.

▸ Gratitude, bring your attention to what ease exists in your life.

▸ Connect with social support.

CHAPTER SUMMARY

Digestive health is fundamental in Ayurveda. Agni, the digestive fire, is the key indicator of our capacity to metabolize what we eat. Ama, the toxic residue from undigested food, is the primary contributor to disease. Stress, both internal and external, significantly impacts agni, and in YoR we aim to bring a relatable aspect to this by presenting it in a more conversational rather than clinical way. Humor helps too; I often think of humor as our much-needed sixth sense! What dosha is driving the bus? Do we tend to under-eat or over-eat? What foods do we crave/resort to? What kind of digestive disturbances do we experience? We now know we must always introduce stress management and spiritual remembrance alongside any attempt to change our food habits. Our kitchen spice rack becomes our first medicine cabinet.

SUGGESTED PRACTICES

Three meals per day with life in between.
Eat your largest meal at lunchtime.
Refrain from eating after 7 pm.

Student Story—One Simple Practice

In addition to codependency, my primary challenge has been my relationship with food (eating disorder). Yoga of Recovery gave me an entirely new construct with which to not only frame my struggles but also actual meaningful tools—beyond external weighing of food and just learning how to say no.

One of the keys in my recovery journey has been establishing daily routines that provide a supportive framework for my healing process, particularly around food. Having regularly spaced mealtimes with ample time to digest, allowing agni to rest, has kept me from binging like I used to. Because my body and mind know I will be taking care of myself when I am naturally hungry again, I don't wait until I am starving to eat, nor am I over-eating to compensate for a meal being skipped or delayed. There is a tangible feeling in my body that I am caring for it as a sacred entity in this one simple practice. There is also less of a chance that I will need to fill or distract the hole that comes around with eating disorders because at the gross, physical level, I know I'm okay.

In addition, incorporating Ayurveda's six tastes has been epic in preventing cravings. Six years ago, I faced a raging sugar addiction that absolutely tortured my mind. In addition to regular mealtimes, making sure that all six tastes are present in every meal—including sweet—greatly reduced my need to grab cookies, ice cream or chocolate after eating (and in between). My mind and body were naturally satisfied. Knocking out the Tamasic junk food also helped raise the prana/energy in my body to where the energy of the empty foods was no longer a match for what my mind and body needed and wanted for sustenance. They were simply energetically incompatible. I also came to realize that a big reason I was craving sweets was heavy consumption of onion and garlic in my meals. Their extreme pungency simply couldn't be balanced by the other tastes; no amount of sweets could establish a feeling of satiation.

Finally, starting an organic fruit and vegetable garden in my backyard has supported my holistic relationship with food. Planting seeds, watching them sprout, tending them, harvesting and consuming or sharing with others helped heal my relationship with food and established a connection with the God-force that was making all of this possible as well as allowing me to ultimately be of joyous service in this world.

Patsy M.

ENDNOTE

1   https://rehabs.com/explore/your-face-on-meth/

Chapter 14

ADDICTIVE TENDENCIES OF THE DOSHAS

A S WE NOW WELL KNOW, Ayurveda says that the first cause of disease is that we forget our true nature is spirit, and the first mask we put on consciousness is the mask of our constitution. We begin to over-identify with our constitution, what I like to call "the doshas driving the bus."

WHEN THE DOSHAS DRIVE THE BUS

When Vata goes out of balance, they seek anything that bolsters their tendency toward busyness and multi-tasking. Then they reach out for things that offer a sense of calm, to decrease the feeling of being scattered that results from excessive activities. Vata more profoundly experiences the rollercoaster effect of addictions. They live for the feeling of being excited, exhilarated, exuberant and can easily be caught in a cycle of impulsively seeking elation, or feeling desperate when they once again feel the pain and insecurity that awaits them at the end of their high. It is generally advised that Vata-dominant constitutional types beware of even the socially acceptable highs, including sugar, caffeine and smoking. Vata requires deep nourishment to sustain their energy, not empty stimulants.

Pitta, the fire type, typically pursues anything that sustains the high level of intensity that they associate with success. They live to advance their feeling of being highly effective and making the world more efficient. They seek out and can easily be caught in a cycle of compulsively seeking anything that makes them feel more powerful and "in charge," and can become very controlling and competitive. There is a drive to win, excel, conquer, succeed, be the best, to place first in the contest of life. They can be prone to perfectionism. They are easily frustrated by mistakes and view them as failures; a reflection of their competitive mindset. Pitta is very attracted to anything that gives them a sense of increased power.

Kapha is generally very amenable to the good life and embraces the feeling of being part of an amicable, tight-knit group. They will often choose things that make them feel at home, comfortable, cozy, on the couch with loved ones and good food. They tend to become more sedentary. Imagine them finding bliss in muscle relaxants and merging with the couch! However, they may also feel the need for stimulants to give them a lift if they feel pushed to live at the pace of our culture. This goes against the grain somewhat as their nature tends to be stable, slow and stoic. It is easy for them to over-eat especially given the large portion sizes now prevailing, especially in the USA.

THE ATTRACTION AND THE PAYBACK

Let's look at the doshas through the lens of what the attraction is to various substances and process behavioral addictions—as well as the payback and damage they inflict. What are we seeking, what are the needs we hope to get met—and what will the damage be? When we can get to the root of understanding this, we can meet our needs in healthier ways, so we aren't left with a feeling of deprivation or exclusion from all the "fun and pleasure" others can partake in.

Alcohol

We drink alcohol for its intoxicating effects; it can temporarily produce feelings of well-being and energy. However, alcohol isn't a stimulant—alcohol is a depressant.

Attraction:

> ▶ Vata may drink to have fun, reduce fear—create confidence and courage, as an ice-breaker in social settings.

▸ Pitta may drink to increase intensity. Generally, alcohol is too hot for the Pitta system, yet Pitta is often drawn to alcohol. Look around an AA meeting, and you'll see a lot of Pitta types. When we forget that our true nature is spirit, we are often drawn to the thing that we think will give us power, which is often the element that is dominant in our constitution; for Pitta, that is fire.

▸ Kapha may use alcohol for stimulation, and to increase the sense of sociability and camaraderie.

Damage/imbalance:

▸ Vata suffers more severely from dehydration, as one of the main and unique qualities of Vata is dryness.

▸ With Pitta, alcohol can seriously overheat the blood and damage the eyes and the liver, as one of the main and unique qualities of Pitta is heat.

▸ For Kapha, the sugar in alcohol can cause swelling, weight gain and a bloated, puffy look from water retention, as one of the main qualities of Kapha is moistness.

Since alcohol is a sugar, it often serves as a substitute for a sugar addiction. In recovery, when we stop drinking alcohol many of us find we gravitate toward use, over-use or even excessive use of sugar. Many alcoholics in recovery—around 95%—have hypoglycemia resulting in anxiety, irritability, sleepiness.

Smoking—Cigarettes and Vaping (also Cannabis when Smoked)

Attraction:

▸ Vata is the element of air and the motor organ is the hands. Oftentimes, Vata types have nervous energy and smoking calms their anxiety, gives them something to do with their hands.

▸ Pitta tends to like the intense feeling of putting more fire into their system. They may smoke to help them control their emotions. They may feel it enhances their image, imagining they look cool or glamorous/masculine.

▸ Kapha likes the stimulation, activating them, alleviating lethargy. They'd also be very happy with a big cigar with an after-dinner drink in a big comfy armchair.

Damage/imbalance:

▸ Vata: Smoking dehydrates and weakens the lungs so there may be a dry cough. It also dehydrates the large intestine, the primary site of Vata, causing constipation.

▸ Pitta: Tobacco is too hot for Pitta leading to inflammatory diseases of the lungs, liver and blood. With Pitta, a strong detox may be required as heat builds up in the body, and wears away the integrity of certain organs and systems governed by Pitta, like the liver and blood.

▸ Kapha: Can experience congestion after giving up smoking; herbal remedies may lessen the effect—these may even be smoked.

All dosha types may be using smoking/vaping as a way to suppress appetite and eat less. Of course, any kind of smoking can cause lung and/or liver cancer, and also result in thyroid issues down the line.

Drugs (Legal and Illegal)

Stimulants (uppers) increase energy and alertness, although the initial high/stimulation they produce is followed by a feeling of exhaustion and/or depression when the drug wears off. We now understand this as excess Rajas (overaction) leading to Tamas (underactivation or downregulation). Examples: Adderall, Ritalin, cocaine, methamphetamine etc.

Depressants (downers) produce an artificial relaxing, sedative effect (Tamas). People turn to them to manage insomnia and anxiety (Rajas). Examples: alcohol, benzodiazepines (Xanax, Klonopin etc.) and barbiturates/tranquilizers (Nembutal/Phenobarbital).

There is such a range of readily available pharmaceuticals in the medicine cabinets of many suburban homes that we can get our hands on almost anything to change our mood whenever we choose. Sometimes they are prescribed and we overdo it, or perhaps we start using someone else's prescribed medications. In YoR we look more closely at the person using the drug: what inner feelings and outer circumstances are they trying to cope with or overcome, rather than the type of drug, or whether it is legal or illegal. I invite you to research for yourself the history of drug criminalization from people like Bill White, who has dedicated his career to researching the history of addiction and treatment and recovery.[1]

We must also be aware that a great debate is occurring around the world about how effective our approach to the drug problem has been. Here is a comment from the American Civil Liberties Union (ACLU):

> More and more ordinary people, elected officials, newspaper columnists, economists, doctors, judges and even the surgeon general of the USA are concluding that the effects of our drug control policy are at least as harmful as the effects of drugs themselves... The best evidence of prohibition's failure is the government's current war on drugs. This war, instead of employing a strategy of prevention, research, education and social programs designed to address problems such as permanent poverty, long term unemployment and deteriorating living conditions in our inner cities, has employed a strategy of law enforcement. While this military approach continues to devour billions of tax dollars and sends tens of thousands of people to prison, illegal drug trafficking thrives, violence escalates and drug abuse continues to debilitate lives.[2]

Attraction:

- ▸ Vata may use drugs to keep them going. Stimulants and amphetamines greatly increase Vata. Regrettably, in low-income populations across the world they are often used to help maintain the pace it takes to make a livable wage. Putting the system in overdrive then produces the need for drugs to calm down, reduce pain and anxiety.

- ▸ Pitta is attracted to drugs that give them an edge, increase their focus, concentration and competitiveness.

- ▸ Kapha can merge into the couch with muscle relaxants.

Damage/imbalance:

- ▸ Vata: Most drugs have a diuretic effect again causing dryness and constipation, but also weakening the kidneys.

- ▸ Pitta: Stimulant drugs aggravate Pitta, damage the eyes and burn out the nervous system.

▶ Kapha: Downers increase Kapha and add more Tamas which greatly imbalances Kapha's qualities of stability and heaviness, increasing them to become obesity and stagnation.

Cannabis

Cannabis as a medicinal herb has muscle relaxant, euphoriant and analgesic effects. It has been used by human beings for many thousands of years. It is mentioned in Ayurveda texts where it is chiefly used for chronic digestive problems for which it can be very effective. Dr. Robert Svoboda speaks about this on YouTube[3]—he notes that any substance/action can always have three possible effects on the body: food, medicine or poison. Cannabis is not a food, or a poison per se. If properly used it can be a good medicine. If not properly used its effects will be more like a slow poison; one that very slowly and often imperceptibly dismantles parts of you because it impedes the flow of prana.

With its increasing legalization in the USA, it will help to understand the reasons some people may fall into overuse through this lens of the addictive tendencies of the doshas. Cannabis is not physically addictive but it is habit-forming, and we know the mind is an addictive mechanism, so it can become addicted to anything.

Attraction:

▶ Vata: May use it to calm down.

▶ Pitta: Allows them to mellow out.

▶ Kapha: May use it to numb out or suppress deep-seated grief.

Damage/imbalance:

▶ Vata: While cannabis is not physically addicting, it is potentially habit-forming especially for Vata dosha which is already prone to addiction. In the short term, it increases Rajas, with its euphoriant effect; in the long term, it creates Tamas.

▶ Pitta: The liver can become chronically congested—there can be subclinical hepatitis, which manifests in irritability, slow wound healing, rashes, yellowing eyes.

▶ Kapha: Low-grade depression, clogs channels and reduces strength of immune system and endurance.[4]

Of course, if it is smoked, we must consider lung and liver cancer. It is also useful to note that because cannabis is fat soluble, it stays in the system longer, up to 30 days, and chronic use can have a negative impact on fertility.

Coffee

Remember the idea that Sattva is relative. Initially it is wise to focus on abstaining from your primary "drug of choice," especially if you are alcohol or chemically dependent. If you have been in recovery for a while and you have problems with sleep, it is wise to consider reducing/giving up coffee, which is Rajasic. Coffee is a nervine, adrenal and cardiac stimulant, often irritating to the intestines, and can be addictive.

Attraction:

▶ Vata: Keeps them busy, multi-tasking.

▶ Pitta: Likes it to increase their focus, drive and intensity.

▶ Kapha: Uses it for its stimulating effects to counteract their sluggishness.

Damage/imbalance:

Many of us (all dosha types) rely on our morning coffee for our bowel movement. However, coffee acts by over-stimulating the gastro-colic reflex and over time the body comes to rely on this over-stimulation, thus creating chronic constipation and making us dependent upon coffee to remain regular.

▶ Vata: Coffee weakens the digestive fire, can cause weight loss, contributes to headaches, palpitations, breathing difficulty, creates dryness in the large intestine.

▶ Pitta: Increases acidity, overheats the blood and liver—leads to inflammation and dryness.

▶ Kapha: Least damaged by moderate coffee use. Its diuretic effect can help Kapha and it can be used occasionally for hypotension, depression and low energy, although there are more beneficial options available and it is preferable to have them prescribed by a practitioner. Overuse can increase the tendency to fibrocystic breast disease.

Food/Disordered Eating/Eating Disorders

We are all dependent on food; however, often we eat to pacify emotions, not to satisfy actual physical hunger. We may feel some sort of lack that we try to fill with tasty food—it could be lack of self-love or self-worth, a sense of emptiness or not being emotionally or spiritually fulfilled. Ayurveda views food also as a manifestation of the five elements; from this comes the six tastes: sweet, sour, salty, pungent, bitter and astringent.

The sweet taste is composed of the elements of earth and water, and makes up around 80% of food, i.e. only 20% of food is dominant in the other tastes. Sweet makes up the bulk of food; it is the most nourishing and building of all the tastes, the aim of Mother Nature being our embodiment. Sweet taste is love-promoting, but often we over-indulge to compensate for a lack of love in our lives.

Vata tends to under-eat, restrict, forget to eat, and skip meals, but this is not sustainable and it can lead to a "feast or famine" mindset, which in turn can lead to anorexia nervosa. We are all "addicted" to food—we must eat, we are dependent on food for our survival, so restriction generally cannot be maintained; hence, bulimia can be another outcome of the over-expression of the Vata dosha impacting our ability to properly nourish ourselves. Vata can also shift from restricted and erratic eating habits into over-eating, which may be their reaction when they realize how empty and famished they feel. They may also resort to eating in a bid to help them calm anxiety, hoping the food will help them feel more grounded, which is unlikely given that they will tend to choose foods that aggravate the Vata qualities, or foods that are difficult to digest due to Vata's disturbed agni.

Vata may be binge-eating in their car, driving from one fast food restaurant to another. Due to the mobile quality of Vata, both under- and over-eating often combine with over-exercising. In the case of under-eating, this causes deep imbalances and can be fatal.

Pitta tends to over-eat under stress. With their strong appetite they usually like to know when they can expect the next meal. They sometimes prioritize task/project completion over eating; however, they generally can't ignore their hunger for too long. When their minds are increasingly disturbed by the effects of Rajas and Tamas they may "aspire" to anorexia as they have a quality of lightness, but due to their strong appetite, they can't sustain restriction for very long and this may lead to purging/bulimia.

Pitta may keep a stash of "bad" food. They will try to eat "right" but if something pushes their stress, they may binge on their secret stash of their stress food choices. Some of these issues may come from them not giving themselves enough quantity of food for the level of hunger they have. Pitta will also tend to over-exercise but it will have a more controlling and calculating feel to it than Vata, who does it more for the love of movement, fun, experience, participation. Pitta is more prone to strict calorie counting and rigid exercise discipline in an effort to overcome their "failure" to control their food intake. They tend to greatly desire control and exhibit hostility toward any impediments. They can often swallow their anger with sweets like ice cream, which they may feel helps them cool down.

Kapha tends to over-eat under stress, just as a matter of course. This is a mistake, as they do not need as much food; they already have a heavy quality and ample quantity of physical substance—earth and water make mud. As the habit of over-eating turns toward a deeper mind-body imbalance, they tend toward emotional over-eating, obesity and depression. They tend to combine this with a more sedentary lifestyle, unlike Vata and Pitta who are more likely to over-exercise. In Rajas, Kapha tend to indulge in sentimentality and are more likely to be found at home, on the couch or very comfortable easy chair, secure in the knowledge that their kitchen cupboards are full of food.

RELATIONSHIP WITH FOOD: FEAR—FUEL—FRIEND

▸ Vata could subconsciously have a "fear" of food. Remember that their survival instinct is to escape, so they should be ready for flight—and lightness is an asset for flight. Also, they experience flatulence, which embarrasses them and makes them more nervous and self-conscious. They also experience bloating, pain and constipation with hard, dry stools. Their confused and clouded minds arrive at the idea that food is the cause of this discomfort so it is better to avoid it. Over-attached to the Vata qualities, they feel rewarded by lightness and mobility.

▸ Pitta may be subconsciously choosing foods that make them a little more sharp and intimidating. We've described their survival instinct as fight and they have strong hunger and anger—the phrase "hangry" describes a Pitta well. They seek out food to "fuel" their already too hot fire, intensity and heat, which they believe sustains their drive and achievement of status and success.

▸ Kapha gravitates to seeing food as their "friend"—it's always there for them and offers them comfort in their melancholy mood and sedentary life at home. When asked to remove certain foods they can feel sad and lonely, especially if it is a food their family favored as they were growing up. It is also related to their survival mode of "tend and befriend"—they aim to maintain secure attachment and closeness through offering food to people. It is a love and peace offering.

Codependence

This is a huge, but important, topic. We just looked at how our dosha dominance can indicate the ways we'll act out with food. Because as babies, food and people are the only things we know, need and are nourished by, and are totally dependent upon, there is a strong possibility that we will also mirror this in our relationships with people:

▸ Vata: Feeling insecure and needy, can develop a "victim" mindset and they may have the idea that the other (their partner, boss, friend, parent, therapist) knows better than them what they need to do. They may need constant verbal reassurance. Abuse as a child creates the ground for a Vata-disturbed psychology.

▸ Pitta: Tends more toward becoming controlling and dominating. They know better than you; they may know better than everyone! Too much conflict or competition in childhood can set this up in the adult years.

▸ Kapha: Tends toward becoming overly attached to others. They feel clingy and perhaps even smothering to be around. Their emotional flavor within unhealthy relationships is "You are their reason for living." Being overly indulged as a child or smothered by parents can play into this.

NON-SUBSTANCE-ORIENTED ADDICTIONS

With substances, we can easily identify the physical and biological impacts on the three doshas. When a person is addicted in other ways, the doshas can still serve to understand the attraction, and of course we must always ask questions to understand why the person pursues a particular outlet. The damages and imbalances they cause to the body are likely to align with the dosha that is causing the attraction.

Gambling

▸ Vata: For fun and excitement.

▸ Pitta: To win/break the game.

▸ Kapha: Motivated by greed.

Shopping

▸ Vata may be an impulsive spender; caught up in fantasy they are more likely to suffer with buyer's remorse once reality sets in, or they may quickly forget they even bought the item, either leaving it to languish in a cupboard, or buying the same item again soon after, being unable to locate the first.

▸ Pitta likes to have the latest technology to advance their drive for efficiency and effectiveness. They are careful shoppers who will do research to find out about product specifications and price comparison.

▸ Kapha loves luxury and possessions. They have a great desire for material comforts which give them a sense of pleasure and security. They tend to accumulate many things and form sentimental attachments to the extent that they feel unable to let go and this can devolve into hoarding the more Tamas takes hold.

THE ONE ADDICTION PROCESS

As we have discussed, there is one addiction process that is alive and well within each of us. While in the past, people in recovery talked about their "drug of choice," today there are so many, it may simply be what's available in various situations. In our culture we have so many options. I heard it described by Cassandra Vieten of the Institute of Noetic Sciences as the "weapons of mass distraction." Many of us resort to a whole range of substances and behaviors to alter how we feel. In YoR we refer to this as our "spread addiction" and use the term "distraction of choice" rather than "drug of choice."

Vata is the most sensitive dosha therefore the most prone to addiction. It controls the nervous system; it is the master dosha. When Deepak Chopra wrote his original book *Overcoming Addictions, The Spiritual Solution*, he mainly addressed the Vata dosha. Most people in active addiction have some kind of Vata imbalance. The daily routines and sensory self-care practices of Ayurveda go a long way in bringing balance to Vata.

What we've looked at in this chapter is the inherent vulnerability that arises when we have a dominance of a particular dosha in our constitution and also, when imbalanced, how the doshas can drive us in certain ways. As we live in habitual forgetfulness of our true nature, we naturally over-identify with our particular version of mind-body, determined by the dominance of particular elements in our constitution. We over-identify with that doshic energy. As a result, we pursue a particular sensation, then often need to medicate that with its opposite to create some fleeting respite.

As we deepen our self-awareness and bring Ayurveda understanding and practices to our recovery and our lives this discipline of self-care totally changes the operating basis of our life. We understand our personal, individual connection with the universal reality. It is such an interesting meeting of the personal with the universal through simple, common sense practices. Being in touch with a deeper self-understanding allows us to be more present and act more intelligently. We have sought change and relief and found it in a host of substances and behaviors but only very briefly. This is expressed so well by Charles T. Tart when he writes, "the relief from suffering that comes from a direct knowledge that the universe is meaningful is far more profound than any other kind of specific, problem-oriented relief."[5] These experiments and experiences and the education they lead us to readies us for more sustainable yet radical change in our being through developing Sattva through the practice of a growth discipline like mindfulness/Yoga and meditation.

CHAPTER SUMMARY

Doshic imbalances are predictable in nature: each dosha tends toward certain modes of thought and action. As a result, they may manifest as addictions to particular substances and behaviors in a misguided attempt to satisfy needs associated with their nature. In bringing an Ayurveda lens to recovery, we can look at which perceived lack or discomfort the dosha is seeking to satisfy, as well as the resulting damage the replacement substances and behaviors cause. When personalized, this allows us to trace a root source of an addictive desire and begin to bring balance by addressing the doshic need(s) underlying it.

SUGGESTED PRACTICE
Abhyanga—Warm Oil Self-Massage

> Abhyanga should be resorted to daily. It wards off old age, exertion and Vata aggravation. It bestows good vision, nourishment to the body, long life, good sleep, good and strong skin...
>
> Aṣṭāṅga Hṛdayam[6]

One unique feature of Ayurveda medicine is its generous use of oils for therapeutic purposes. Abhyanga is the anointing of the body with warm, often herbal oils.

Set aside around 15 minutes for self-massage each day. Beginning at the extremities and working toward the middle of your body, massage the oil* into your body, using long strokes on the limbs and circular strokes on the joints. Massage the abdomen and chest in broad, clockwise, circular motions. On the abdomen, follow the path of the large intestine, moving up on the right side of the abdomen, then across, then down on the left side. Do this with patience, perhaps repeating an affirmation about self-love and self-care. In YoR we call this our boundary work, where we take time to lovingly tend to our skin, the boundary where we feel and meet the world. This is a powerful therapy for mind-body.

Visit www.yogaofrecovery.com for more information on what oils to use, contraindications and practical advice regarding towels and laundry.

Student Story—I Got This!

I was raised in a dysfunctional, alcoholic family in the Midwest. It was painful and uncomfortable on all levels, and I started drinking at around the age of 12. At 25 I moved to California, I married at 30, had a baby—and continued to drink until I was 40-something.

On January 1, 2000, I began a life of sobriety, after spending the night in jail. For the next 15 years I stayed sober through the 12 Steps; I became a Yoga teacher and read all the self-help books. I thought my life was okay. Now that I look back, though, life was definitely not okay. I was physically, emotionally and spiritually sick.

In March 2010 shit hit the fan; my mom passed away, and that started a downhill spiral that dropped me to my knees. Within months, my marriage of 25 years ended, I moved into a small house and felt lost and detached. Soon after, my best friend lost her seven-year struggle to cancer, my older sister passed away due to complications in surgery and my 14-year-old dog died. Then my daughter said I was crazy and told me she needed a break from me.

I was a mess! Broken, sick, lonely, angry.

Whenever I'm in a dark place Durga's Yoga of Recovery teachings pull me back to the light. With her help, I found Dr. Suhas, an Ayurveda doctor in Santa Cruz, and did a Panchakarma that involved cleaning up my diet and committing to self-care practices like Yoga and meditation. I soon pulled myself up from the floor, brushed the dust off, wiped away my tears and got a tattoo that says, "I got this!"

Today, happy and healthy, I teach YoR at Kaiser Hospital in northern California to a group of amazing people who have stepped into the world of sobriety. I share my stories of hurt and healing with them in hopes that somehow my story will inspire theirs, and in hopes that they too will find peace through practice.

Linda B.

ENDNOTES

1   www.williamwhitepapers.com
2   www.aclu.org/other/against-drug-prohibition
3   Svoboda, R. (2021) *An Ayurvedic Perspective on Cannabis: 5 Minutes with Dr Robert* [Channel: Dr. Robert Svoboda]. www.youtube.com/watch?v=WvKhYTSGO9E
4   I am grateful for the contribution of Akalananda Ma, Alandi Ayurveda Clinic in Boulder Colorado, to my knowledge through her very helpful educational articles (www.alandi-ashram.org).
5   Miller, D.P. (2002) *News of a New Human Nature: The Best Features & Articles on the New Spirituality*. Napa, CA: Fearless Books, p. 130.
6   Welch, C. (2016) *Dinacaryā* (3rd edn) [ebook]. https://drclaudiawelch.com/shop/books/dinacharya-changing-lives-through-daily-living/

Chapter 15

COUNSELING THE DOSHA TYPES

IN THIS CHAPTER, we are going to look at the psychological disorders that the doshas are prone to, due to their natural tendencies when the mind is dominated by the Rajas and Tamas gunas. We will also look at the best approach to guide each dosha type back toward Sattva, through self-regulation, self-care and routine, sharing with others and finding community. This is a very helpful perspective as we have many different approaches and opinions about recovery across different fields, and concern has been voiced over the "tough love" measures that some fear too easily become force and indoctrination. Whereas some people need gentleness and more of a coaching approach, this would be too soft a method in some cases or at different stages with the same person or in certain areas of their lifestyle choices.

The Ayurveda idea of constitution and the tendencies of imbalance in the doshas on the psychological level can indicate how to counsel different temperaments in more appropriate ways. As we have all three doshas within us we may want to consider the following information as a guide in how to work with our own specific temperament in a healthier way, bearing in mind our growth/evolution journey through the lens of the gunas—moving to Sattva through the higher aspect of Rajas, from the diseased state that is Tamas. David Frawley's book *Ayurveda and the Mind* discusses this in detail. Much of what follows in this chapter comes from this book, rephrased and reorganized.

No matter the doshic imbalance, we saw in Chapter 4 on the gunas that those in the state of Tamas need more strict supervision, and require attendance in a fairly rigorous disciplined daily schedule, because left to their own devices they will too easily sink back into old destructive habits.

A well-prepared intervention, a thoroughly researched detox in an inpatient facility followed by an inpatient or outpatient rehabilitation program, according to the patient's needs, and crucially—yet regrettably—the ability to access this level of care. This is likely to be the stage where medically prescribed pharmaceuticals may play a role in the solution, hopefully carefully monitored with a view to this not necessarily becoming the complete long-term solution.

Those who are more in Rajas will often have good intentions but may find it hard to steadily implement changes on their own; they find it benefits them to opt for some accountability and group support. They may also find difficulty in completing what they embark on for various reasons like distractions, time demands, changes of heart, deciding some other activity is preferred etc. I think we can all recognize areas where we are in need of the support of others and hopefully we've felt the benefits of asking for and accepting all the different levels of support that are available to us: Yoga classes, Yoga therapy sessions, peer-supported recovery groups, work with sponsors and sponsees, Ayurveda consultations and one-to-one psychotherapy etc.

In YoR we continuously honor our personal needs within each stage of our recovery process from the perspective of the gunas:

- Tamas—we need more strict supervision.

- Rajas—we do better by opting for accountability and group participation and support.

- Sattva—we're more able to self-initiate our wellness practices but still show up for group participation as we recognize the value of service and satsang.

HOW TO WORK WITH VATA

Vata constitutional types are prone to:

- excessive thinking and worry

- feeling nervous, anxious and afraid

- being overly sensitive, excessively reactive

- taking things too personally

- premature, inappropriate action

- being ungrounded, spaced out, unrealistic

- insomnia.

High Vata in the mind:

- Can be overenthusiastic and excited (this seldom lasts), followed by quickly quitting or getting distracted.

- Expect too much too soon.

- Ungrounded, hard to pin down, can be **deceptive**.

- Often have negative attitude about themselves.

- May have a more negative attitude about their disease than it actually merits.

- Possible hypochondriac, may be seeking attention and sympathy (adverse childhood experiences can reinforce that this is the way we receive attention).

- Happy to receive advice but inconsistent in the follow through.

Vata imbalance primary in the mind:
Fear, alienation, possible nervous breakdown, tremors, palpitations, restlessness, rapid mood shifts, wrong imaginings, hallucinations, delusions including hearing voices, ranting and rambling (essentially incoherent), may begin to live in their thoughts and confuse their thoughts with reality.

Extreme signs of Vata imbalance include: bipolar (formerly called manic depression), schizophrenia.

Causes of high Vata in the mind:
Like increases like. With qualities of light, dry and mobile, the Vata dosha tends toward flight. They tend to believe change is the solution; they experience restlessness.

- Drugs and stimulants aggravate Vata (caffeine, sugar and stronger substances—alcohol and substance use disorders).

▸ Disturbing sensations (true with all doshas): over-exposure to media (news, rapidly changing scenes on screens), loud music, noise (the element of ether—Vata governs sound).

▸ Variable appetite—insufficient food and irregular eating can aggravate Vata. As mentioned in Chapter 13 they can tend to eat foods that aggravate the Vata dosha even further by favoring dry, light, cold, raw foods.

▸ Stress, fear and anxiety provoke Vata.

▸ Violence and trauma cause hurt and the tendency to withdraw or even dissociate.

▸ Neglect and abuse in childhood create a predisposition for a Vata-disturbed psychology.

Vata Counseling Profile

▸ Requires time and patience to change.

▸ Need to calm both mind and heart: aim for slow, steady growth.

▸ Counteract Vata's tendency of being caught up in their problems, but not actually doing something about them. They like to talk about their challenges, but this may not be very helpful. We let them know we hear them, remind them that they are loved and supported.

▸ They may constantly seek verbal reassurance, but it doesn't help for them to talk incessantly about their problems. We offer validation while encouraging them toward practical things that are to be implemented in a consistent manner.

▸ Set boundaries. Vata tends to think "you know better than them what they should do." If we buy into this, we encourage dependency.

▸ Including daily Abhyanga is the main way to pacify Vata through physical means. Vata's primary element is air which governs the sense of touch, skin and hands. Abhyanga oils are heavy, warming and grounding which are the opposite qualities to Vata which is cold, light, dry and mobile; therefore, it is very nourishing for all Vata-disturbed psychological symptoms.

▸ Find ways to **encourage Vata to stick with it**.

Treat Vata Like a Flower

▸ Approach them with warmth, calmness and determination.

▸ Let them feel your support without allowing dependency.

▸ Emphasize action rather than thought—steady action rather than seeking quick results.

▸ Comprehensive routine is important: across the timeline of the day. It's important that they are regularly grounded throughout the day with timed daily self-care practices and self-remembrance.[1]

HOW TO WORK WITH PITTA

Pitta constitutional types are prone to:

▸ strong self-control, but can be self-centered and antisocial

▸ mind can become narrow and contentious—angry, aggressive, hostile

▸ overly critical type who finds fault with everyone around them

▸ tendency to blame others

▸ see enemies everywhere

▸ on guard, ready for a fight

▸ they like to investigate and debate but may get drawn into conspiracy theories—viewing things with suspicion—an incriminating rather than discriminating perspective.

High Pitta in the mind:

▸ Blame and think they know best.

▸ Most disturbed by conflict with other people which they exaggerate or exacerbate.

- ▸ Drama of interpersonal struggle colors their minds and emotions.

- ▸ Prone to be at war with themselves.

- ▸ Can torment themselves with unrealistically high standards. Pittas are ever achieving and they expect to see this in others.

- ▸ They like authority and are impressed by credentials.

- ▸ Tend to be aggressive, critical, sometimes contentious and **destructive**.

- ▸ May question the therapist's qualifications, like to tell people what they should do for them, respond with anger and criticism (if things don't go their way).

Pitta imbalance primary in the mind:

Anger, frustration, agitation, irritability, possible violent behavior, domineering, authoritarian or fanatical.

Extreme signs of Pitta imbalance include: paranoid delusions, delusions of grandeur or psychosis.

Causes of high Pitta in the mind:

Like increases like. With qualities of heat, instability and light, the Pitta dosha tends toward fight. They tend to believe control is the solution; they experience irritability.

- ▸ Exposure to violence and aggression (including media, politics).

- ▸ Hot, spicy food.

- ▸ Sexual frustration, excessive anger and ambition.

- ▸ Disturbing sensations: strong lights and bright colors and sensations.

- ▸ Too much conflict/competition during childhood creates a predisposition for a Pitta-disturbed psychology.

Pitta Counseling Profile

- ▶ More receptivity is encouraged; less judgment.

- ▶ Use kind, firm behavior; do not allow yourself to get drawn into their competitive dramas.

- ▶ Pitta has fire of the mind: sharp intellect, critical insight. We need to help them see how their problems reside in their own behavior reactions. Teach them right use of discrimination and self-reflection.

- ▶ Approach with tact and diplomacy: they do not like to be told what to do. In Rajas, they like to be in control. It is important to appeal to their natural intelligence because opposing them will not help them grow.

- ▶ In alcoholic homes, there is a tendency toward black and white thinking. We need to help them seek a balanced view, become considerate of others and more diplomatic in their actions. Encourage them to see that other people are doing the best they can given their situation and resources. This can be a wake-up call for Pitta because they tend toward "my way is the right way."

Treat Pitta Like a Friend

- ▶ They like forming alliances; they work well with people they respect.

- ▶ Once they know what to do, they are usually the best of all three doshas at implementing and following through on behavioral changes. They can sometimes go to the extreme, becoming fanatical and rigid.

- ▶ In YoR we advise "never pet a Pitta!" Generally, they will bristle if they are spoken to in too much of a soft, reassuring tone—too much of a "there, there now" approach. That is well received by Vata types but Pitta can be disturbed by this; they can feel as though you think they do not know what they are doing. It is best to ally with a Pitta. Introduce the suggestion and once they get on board, be willing to step back and concur with the great idea they've come up with to solve their dilemma—let it be their idea.

- ▶ With Pitta, it's important to **encourage moderation.**[2]

HOW TO WORK WITH KAPHA

Kapha constitutional types are prone to:

▶ the least psychological problems

▶ less likely to express their problems, especially by resorting to anti-social behavior; they like to stay in the comfort and familiarity of their own home—so their reactions aren't as publicly disruptive as Vata and Pitta types

▶ tend to be shy, tend to want to only be around people they know well (stranger danger)

▶ attachment

▶ greed—want material wealth, possessions

▶ easily discontented.

High Kapha in the mind:

▶ Blocked mind, clouded senses, mental dullness, congestion and poor perception (like a mudslide).

▶ Prone to addictions and depression.

▶ Lack of drive and motivation, which can lead to **depression**, sorrow, clinging.

The description of the stress reaction of Kapha in YoR is "tend and befriend." When they are in distressing circumstances, they will do what they need to do to pacify the threat. Our addictiveness is largely a relational problem and mostly we are unable to run away or fight with those who we don't get on with or who bully, threaten or dominate us, yet ultimately it is our relationship with our own self that is dysfunctional. Kapha represents the part in us that survives by "hunkering down." This is the part of us that tends to camouflage in order to fit in and not rock the boat. It has a lot to do with how we learn to reflect our immediate environment which is an instinctual survival mechanism of our subconscious mind, our herd mentality. In essence we lose our identity, we are out of touch with our own needs, desires and feelings as we continuously try to do what we *think* others want or expect of us.

Kapha imbalance primary in the mind:

▸ Slow to act, hard to change, resorts to a resigned complacency.

▸ Inertia and stagnation bogs them down.

▸ Oftentimes they don't want to be disloyal to their family, friends or teachers.

▸ Kapha holds memories for a long time and what they think was recent can be actually ten or 15 years ago whereas the other two doshas go through things at a more rapid rate.

▸ Most of their problems come from excess emotionality, which can be changed by developing higher love and detachment.

Extreme signs of Kapha imbalance include: The mind can become incapable of abstract, objective, rational thinking. Everything relates to their limited personal field of experience. They are prone to be passive and this can progress to them feeling so dependent they become child-like; they just want to be taken care of, perhaps even becoming unable to take care of themselves. They may seek comfort and consolation from their therapist, but this should not be encouraged as it is partly their sentimentality about their condition that helps them sustain it. They may need/desire a care home where someone can help take care of them when they are unable to take care of themselves.

Causes of high Kapha in mind:

▸ too much sleep

▸ daytime sleep

▸ lack of exercise

▸ too much sugar or oily food

▸ excess pleasure, enjoyment, attachment to life

▸ emotional problems will combine with Kapha's physical proclivities and worsen that heavy feeling

▸ their tendency is to return to old habits, especially those favored by their family and friends

▸ being overly indulged as a child, overly cosseted or emotionally smothered may lead to Kapha-disturbed psychology.

Kapha Counseling Profile

▸ Treat Kapha with more firmness and frequency:

  – Approach with more **firmness**; it takes determination and consistency in order for them to be made acutely aware of the problem, perhaps even a sense of force.

  – Need more **frequent** appointments and more constant interchange to get them started—coax them out of their complacency.

▸ Needs to be stimulated and perhaps even sometimes shocked.

▸ Kapha types have difficulty discussing their problems; they are comfortable with only a few close family and friends and tend to have a feeling of "stranger danger." They only learn to trust you and let you in over time, but once you are accepted, they tend to have "forever" connections.

▸ As they are less direct, listen closely to really assess where they are stuck or suffering.

▸ It helps for them to have an exercise buddy/commitment—here we capitalize on their tendency to "tend and befriend." Get them started with some easy or moderate exercise. If you assign too challenging a task at the outset, they just want to stop; but once they get started they can then access the strength, endurance and power within themselves and feel stronger after the first five to ten minutes, when the blood and breath start to move.

▸ The initiation and implementation of new behaviors is very challenging but once they start, they can continue steadily. They can be as easily accustomed to a healthy flow versus an unhealthy flow. The challenge is the transition. Moving a Kapha is like moving a boulder—it is difficult to get the momentum going, but once started, it moves more easily.

▸ Encourage Kapha to go the extra mile, do more than they think they can do.[3]

BUTTERFLY, BULL OR TORTOISE?

In Ayurveda, we sometimes compare each dosha to an animal. Vata is like a butterfly or bee, going swiftly from one flower to another, always on the move. Pitta is like the bull; it sees its desired destination, puts its head down and charges directly to the finish line. Kapha are like tortoises, slow and steady; when things do not go well, they shrink back into their shells—withdrawn and silent. They don't say much, argue or become aggressive.

These ideas above give us a starting place for how to work with each doshic type. What we learn applies to working firstly with our own natures and then others. We want to know when to treat ourselves like a flower and when like a friend. We have to know when to be gentle with ourselves and when to challenge ourselves, being firm and perhaps forcing ourselves to do things we tend to avoid—like asking for help. The answers may change based on circumstances—especially what level of "addictiveness" we have reached and the object(s) of our acting out.

FAITH, COMPASSION AND DETACHMENT

Remember Our True Nature

Our true nature is spirit, eternal beings. Forgetting this is the primordial cause of disease. We come forth into this physical manifestation and naturally over-identify with our body-mind "container" which is composed of the five elements (ether, air, fire, water, earth) operating as the three biological forces/doshas (Vata, Pitta, Kapha).

Remembrance of the self/source is part of the spiritual solution to our addictiveness and the resultant stress of separation it brings. A consistent meditation practice helps a great deal (and this is a recommendation of the 11th Step of the 12-Step programs). In YoR, we also emphasize the creation of a habit of inner resourcing (Chapter 1), connecting with a place within that is at ease, peaceful, calm and secure. These practices give us a refuge, so we can step back from the tumultuous waves of Rajas, and the drag of the undercurrent of Tamas. Our inner connection becomes like a safe port in the storm for us, where we can remember and reconnect with a deeper truth and refresh our energy to step out and again meet and greet the world from a more centered, calm place.

See with the Heart's Eye

We have a tendency in Ayurveda to talk about the constitutional type and this serves a purpose, to an extent, but we can over-identify and even start to stereotype and identify too superficially. As individuals, members of family and community, practitioners and perhaps 12-Step sponsors or professional counselors, we have to remember that we are all five-element beings so it is important not to interpret ourselves and others too narrowly as one particular dosha "type." We all have all three doshas within us, so it is helpful to rec-ognize all three as tendencies within us, although people may pattern their reactions strongly in one direction in general, or more so at a certain time of life or in particular situations. At heart, the primary way to move beyond emotional distress is to increase Sattva. This helps us build dispassion and discrimination (Vairagya and Viveka) so we make better self-care choices more naturally. We become good custodians of our mind-body system.

It is important to keep the vision of who we are in our balanced state and to see others with the heart's eye, remembering them at their more balanced level, especially when they have forgotten. This means that "Namaste" is the guiding principle of Ayurvedic counseling: honoring the light in ourselves and recognizing that same light in others.

Pause, then Respond

YoR suggests that a core part of long-term sobriety and emotional stability is creating *pause* space to prevent us from always being in Rajas—stress reac-tive/overactivation mode, which leads to Tamas, downregulated, exhausted, underactivated. With practice, support and encouragement this pause can bring us to a more appropriate, present moment, spontaneous response, rather than constantly recycling our old reactions—one definition of insanity is doing the same thing over and over again expecting different results.

The pause allows us to find a way to practice a Sattvic response or, as Swami Sivananda would say, an opportunity to practice a virtue rather than a vice.[4] In the pause, we ask: In this moment, does this particular situation require me to be more light-hearted, creative and inventive (Sattvic Vata); or would all be better served by sharing vision, discipline and leadership (Sattvic Pitta); or is the role of patience, kindness and nurturing required (Sattvic Kapha)?

There is no one protocol that works for everyone. When confronted with someone who is controlling, validate them and encourage them to develop a way to be heard by others. Recognize and acknowledge who they'd be in their Sattvic manifestation. Do our best to remind and coach others toward that.

Settle into this basic truth: we do not have the personal power to change anyone other than our own self. Sattva is the ability to respond in the moment to what is needed. We do not set our sights on changing the person in front of us; we set our intention on changing our own response to those around us. As we communicate with others our intention and practice is to be the most conscious self that we can be in the moment.

We know it is our own perception that creates our reality—as we find that space to pause then respond, rather than react or resist, our reality changes. Regular meditation trains us in creating more space for the pause, so we can free ourselves from being controlled by, and at the mercy of, our reactions to our environment and the people around us. Our aim is to increasingly meet ourselves and others with unconditional positive regard and acceptance.

CHAPTER SUMMARY

One size does not fit all in Ayurveda. There are different manifestations of these addictions. We need ongoing support through all the stages of the recovery process—so there is an adaptation that needs to occur. The predominant guna that is active in our life, or our client's life, helps to show the approach we'll need in order to be successful. There is no one protocol that works for everyone. In order to offer support in the most effective way, an understanding of the psychological disposition of the predominant dosha(s) makes a difference in ours and our client's ability to relate to the guidance and be able to implement and sustain change. Most importantly, we combine this knowledge with a compassionate presence (Sattva) that sees beyond definitions, diagnoses and types, and remembers that it is the idea of separation itself that is the root cause of our suffering.

Becoming a good counselor is very similar to being on a spiritual path—the willingness to pay attention and recognize our intention from the deeper source, which is spirit. We have described the clear light of consciousness coming through us steadily as Sattva. This manifests through Vata as creativity, enthusiasm and artistic flair; for Pitta, the ability to lead and guide; and for Kapha, kindness and nurturing. What we can experiment with is to choose our response to any situation from these descriptions rather than coming at it from our entrenched personality pattern—which often stems from our own stress reactions or repeated inappropriate coping mechanisms around adverse experiences and trauma. When confronted with someone who is controlling, we can aim to validate them and encourage them to develop a way to be heard by others. Our work is to recognize and acknowledge what is best in the person, and remind them of that often.

The ACA version of the Serenity Prayer can be of great assistance to remind us of the one person we have the power to change: "Spirit, grant me the serenity to accept the people I cannot change, courage to change the one I can and the wisdom to know that one is me."[5]

SUGGESTED PRACTICE
Administer Nasal Oil (Nasya)

Nasya is an oil or herbal oil that is either applied to the inside of the nostrils, or sniffed in through them. It benefits the head, face, hair, vision, smell, hearing, stiff neck, headache, facial paralysis, lockjaw, rhinitis, migraine, head tremors, veins, joints, ligaments and tendons of the skull. We can use warm, untoasted sesame oil or herbal oil. It is wise, again, to check with your health care practitioner to determine what would be best for you. I like Super Nasya Oil from the Ayurvedic Institute and Calamus Ghee from Rich Fisher (see www.yogaofrecovery.com for links and guidance on how to administer the oil into the nostrils).

Student Story—Peeling Away the Layers

I have a lot of different teachers I turn to in my journey, but Durga was my first teacher, and the teacher I will always attribute all of my successes to. Hers is the voice I hear in my head as I navigate through life.

I wasn't always the most balanced student. I think I was even a difficult student for her at first, especially in early recovery, but she has always guided me with compassion and love to help me "peel away the layers of the onion" to bring me deeper and deeper into connection to my true self. Now, Ayurveda is my main medical system and has helped me overcome all of the other addictions that have crept up on me throughout my recovery—nicotine, both

over- and under-eating habits, codependency and love addiction. Most importantly, all symptoms of my PTSD from sexual violence are completely gone.

In Yoga of Recovery, Durga explains the deep philosophies and concepts
of Yoga and Ayurveda in a way that is down to earth and approachable. I have
now taken this course about five times and each time, another of my addictive
"acting out" behaviors falls away. She is also the person who first brought me to
India for Panchakarma, a month-long deep Ayurveda cleanse which introduced
me to the life I am leading today.

Tarini R.

ENDNOTES

1   Frawley, *Ayurveda and the Mind*, pp. 154–168.
2   ibid.
3   ibid.
4   Swami Sivananda has written numerous books which you can download for free from
     www.dlshq.org
5   ACA, *Adult Children of Alcoholics/Dysfunctional Families*, p. 424.

Chapter 16

DETOXIFICATION OF THE MIND

DETOXIFYING THE MIND IS VERY IMPORTANT in Ayurveda as healing, coming back to wholeness, depends on our ability to tune with our physical and mental needs, and with our unique sense of self and how we interact with others and our environment in order to get our needs met. Remember it is the effect of the gunas of Rajas and Tamas on the mind that create disease and suffering; think of it as the force of projection and veiling preventing us from accessing the natural power of an integrated mind.

How do you detox the mind? First we stop taking the toxins in and start fasting from the mental impressions. This first step is to either completely avoid, or at least limit, taking in that which causes imbalance within us. This is one of the main areas of debate in the addiction field and also a major difficulty for the individual who desires to achieve abstinence while still experiencing stress that triggers cravings for the things we are trying to avoid.

MEDITATION

The ability to maintain abstinence from something we still feel we desire, need or crave requires establishing a greater ability to rein in the mind and senses and this is greatly aided by the daily practice of asana and pranayama. However, as we are unable to protect ourselves from all negative impressions, we need to develop the power of our deeper intelligence to develop both detachment and discernment/discrimination. This is one of the main goals of our physical Yoga practices: to help us calm our turbulent energy so we can commit to a consistent daily meditation practice. There are many resources to support us in settling into a meditation practice. I personally like the regularly offered free 21-day Meditation Challenges offered from the Chopra center.[1]

INNER RESOURCE/BODY SENSING

In YoR, we introduce connection to the centered state of calm and inner awareness through the practice of Inner Resource Meditation. We have already been introduced to the practice in Chapter 1. Let's look more deeply at its importance and its mechanisms.

It's important to do regular body-sensing and breath-sensing check-ins to become more aware of the sensations in our body. And why does this matter? As we tune in more regularly to our body sensations, locating where our thoughts or emotions are manifesting in the body, we can actually allow our mind to gently rest with that sensation, begin to meet and greet it, rather than reacting or resisting it by reaching for external distractions. We begin to actually feel our feelings, not just think about them or avoid them. By practicing body and breath sensing we can slowly detach from the ego mind's constant narrative—the stories in our mind that repeat on us incessantly. As we locate the story as sensation in the body and meet, greet and welcome it we start to notice how transient sensation really is; it is quite hard to hold on to a physical sensation for any length of time, without it morphing and changing. In this practice, if any sensation feels overwhelming to us we again take refuge in our Inner Resource which is a felt sensation of calm and ease that we can access instantly especially with repeated practice. This ability to find a place within us where we can rest at ease allows us to find some composure and return to feel the sensation when we feel ready.

We no longer have to push away our feelings or rely on something external. Our ability to balance these pairs of opposites exists within us on a more subtle level as well as outside us through the appropriate food and herbs etc. We can allow ourselves to be the witness of all the sensations that are coming and going and rest in awareness, which is the truth of our deepest, innermost nature of consciousness, the observer. We come to know our mind as an instrument. When done regularly, we can begin to adopt the tools required to balance our mental field. This happens naturally as we learn not to push our thoughts and emotions away. By allowing and just paying attention to body sensations, we realize they are temporary. Body and breath are in the now; the mind will continue with its story. Remember, the world is not how it is; it is how we see it. If we are emotionally dis-regulated, our world will be too.

This Too Shall Pass

This is important for those in recovery: coming to the awareness that our thoughts and emotions are an embodied experience, and therefore transient; what is constant is our ability to witness that which comes and goes. 12-Step recovery programs have a slogan "This too shall pass"—body sensing is the embodiment of this slogan. For instance, we become able to feel into our fear, realizing that each thought/emotion also contains its opposite. When we observe this with our full intention and attention, we begin to embody the emotional part of the detoxification.

Most of us are familiar with the idea of avoiding certain foods to help detoxify the physical body. This is also applicable to the "objects of our affections" in relation to sensory impressions. When we draw back from full-on sense participation we create time and space for deeply cleansing Yogic practices of meditation and self-inquiry. In YoR, we investigate the paths of Yoga through a course called "Healing the Habits that Bind: The 6 Tenets of Yoga of Recovery" (see www.yogaofrecovery.com for details of this offering).

Panchakarma

Ayurveda and Yoga work on all three levels of our manifestation: physical, subtle and causal (the karmic seed that brought us here). On the physical level, we focus on the type and quality of food, regular meals, eating only when we are hungry, awareness of portion size, choosing sustainable food, cooking with love, paying attention to eating quietly and with gratitude. We can also make use of herbs, asana and exercise.

In addition, Ayurveda offers a deep detoxification process known as Panchakarma. YoR runs a Panchakarma retreat each year, inviting students to India to undergo a deep cleanse which involves a light diet, specific herbs and body treatments. First there is a preparatory period, followed by the actual eliminatory procedures, and then comes the rebuilding phase. It takes time to coax ama (toxins) and imbalanced doshas back to the GI tract—that's where it originates (as undigested foods) before it relocates into tissues and organs.

We bring it back to the "central office of the doshas"—those sites of accumulation (Kapha in the stomach, Pitta in the small intestine and Vata in the large intestine) for elimination. The body releases toxins through the urine, feces and sweat. This process, when done thoroughly, with proper medical care and rest, re-establishes metabolic and hormonal balance. It also takes time; hence, for the YoR Panchakarma trip in India we require at least three to four weeks.

While the specific details of Panchakarma are beyond the scope of this book, it helps to appreciate this aspect of Ayurveda: that while we can make great strides in achieving balance through self-healing, we can also submit ourselves to professional care and receive physical treatment. It is reassuring to know that we can ask for help and be the recipient of care. Many of us do need help in repairing the damage done. It takes time and commitment; we must be willing to be patient and go within. This is not so much a social or a learning retreat; it is a retreat of quietude and letting go. Only those for whom it seems appropriate are invited to attend. During that retreat, in the safety of the womb-like conditions of the loving and gentle care we receive in the clinic, we dive deeper into emotional detoxification through dyad co-meditation work.

TRAUMA IS PSYCHOLOGICAL AMA

The main aim of Panchakarma is to eliminate ama from the body to restore its proper function and health. There is also psychological ama. I see the word "AMA" embedded in the word trauma—trAuMA. Remember ama literally means "that which harms or weakens." Ayurveda is clear that we need proper digestive fire to digest both physical substances and mental impressions.

Many of us have been exposed to trials and tribulations we have not yet been able to completely digest. This is especially true for anyone who has experienced adverse childhood/community/climate experiences or early childhood trauma, and we are now well aware that this is often a causative factor in addictions and mental health issues. We need help to shift out of these old belief systems—out of the Tamas. Ama and Tamas are really what trauma is—on all levels—physical, mental, emotional and causal (i.e. it is part of our karma).

Addiction is a complex multi-layered problem that is not solved simply by putting down our "drug of choice." When we put that down, we are going to be left to face the pre-existing painful condition that led to the use in the first place. Studies show how much ACEs contribute to these underlying issues.[2] Abuse, abandonment and neglect in early childhood set up a tendency toward a Vata imbalance. We use the term PTSD, "*Post*" Traumatic Stress Disorder. The first word is "post" because it indicates the past—and *now*, our best chance at health is to live within present-moment awareness. Tamas and ama can form a toxic blanket that seems to protect us from the outside world by letting us remain disconnected from our own true feelings and needs.

HOW DO WE CHANGE THE PAST?

What long-term recovery and emotional sobriety require is a continuum of care within a supportive community. True healing is a transformational process. How do we change the past? Here, I turn to a truly beautiful and empowering perspective on Ayurveda daily routines from Claudia Welch.[3]

> There is a principle accepted by Eastern medical traditions, including Ayurveda, pertaining to the relationship between microcosms and macrocosms. Here is how Caraka, an ancient sage of Ayurveda describes it:
>
> The individual is not different from the universe.
>
> All natural phenomena in the universe exist in the individual.
>
> Everything that exists in the macrocosm exists in the microcosm, and the reverse is true as well: everything that exists in the microcosm exists in the macrocosm.
>
> The Law of Macrocosm and Microcosm is a fundamental principle in Ayurveda that can have profound implications. There is the cycle of life, from conception to birth, childhood, middle age, old age, death and—if we accept the idea of reincarnation—to rebirth.
>
> In relation to dinacarya... we can be particularly interested in the relationship between the 24-hour cycle microcosm and the macrocosm of the life-cycle of a human being. In the morning when we wake, our senses and consciousness transition from sleep to daily reality, in a similar way as when our senses awaken when we are born and transition from life within the womb to life outside of it. We become more active in the middle part of the day, as the

middle portion of our lives tend to be more ambitious and active, and then we slow down in the evening, preparing for sleep, as we slow in old age, preparing for our ultimate transition to death. We could say this, then: that early morning roughly corresponds to pregnancy, birth and early childhood, morning corresponds to later childhood, midday to midlife, and late afternoon through twilight equates to old age or the twilight of life. Nightfall signifies death and, if we accept reincarnation (not a necessity to benefit from the practice of dinacarya), nighttime would correlate with the mysteries encountered by the un-embodied soul between lifetimes.

If the macrocosm of our lifetime can be affected by the microcosm of one day, it follows that it is important *how* we spend that day. The sages who first delivered the precepts of Ayurveda were well aware of this and outlined guidelines for a healthy dinacarya; guidelines we can adjust according to seasons and our various needs and constitutions.

While we may have little or no control over the grander cycles of ages, the seasons or even our present lifetime, we do have an opportunity each day to take advantage of a new day. And how we spend the microcosm of a day may affect the macrocosm of a lifetime.

It is of particular interest to note that, while general life principles are given as guidelines to live our daily lives, the bulk of specific directions for dinacarya [from the classical Ayurveda texts] are geared towards a morning routine, from waking sometime between 4 am and dawn, to meditating, grooming, exercising and bathing. All this takes place before breakfast. From breakfast onward we are left to our discretion, to apply ethical living to our particular needs and patterns. Before we look at the rest of the day, let's consider why so much emphasis is given to the early morning routine.

I think the healing comes from the potential we can tap from the relationship between early morning and early human development, introduced above. Let us explore this a little more.

If indeed the early morning time period relates to pregnancy and birth, we would suspect that there would be similarities between the two. And indeed there are. One striking similarity is that both times are governed by Vata—a biological force associated with periods of change, transition, movement, the nervous system, formation of neural pathways and all mental and physical movement.

If dawn relates to birth, pre-dawn hours would relate to pregnancy. It would stand to reason that damaging or healing influences on Vata would be particularly significant during both the early morning hours and during early human development, when we were in the womb, being born, or experiencing our first months or years of life.

Both Ayurveda and Western medicine recognize that what happens to us in utero and early in life is crucial in forming lifelong patterns and rhythms, because our organs, tissues, emotional patterns and proclivities are developed during this time. Patterns established during this time are often difficult—sometimes thought impossible—to change. Trauma during these critical formative stages aggravates Vata and often creates khavaigunyas—challenge [weak/vulnerable] areas—in various organs or systems or proclivities. Sometimes these can have a negative impact on our physical, mental and emotional patterns throughout our lives.

For example, one person may feel a vague, free-floating sense of anxiety for her entire life. Another may have always had a weak digestive system or impaired cognitive abilities. Still another may find herself unable to have healthy intimate relationships. Often there is a sense of hopelessness about changing these tenacious patterns.

Whenever we see a pattern that dates back as far as we can remember in our lives, we can guess it has its inception in conception, pregnancy, birth or very early childhood. I frequently see patients with difficult lifelong physical or emotional patterns resulting from trauma suffered in utero, during birth or in childhood. Often they feel a sense of hopelessness about changing these patterns. Sometimes we are even taught in Ayurveda or other medical modalities that these conditions are impossible to change.

Could it really be true that something we had no control over as a developing fetus, or an infant, will negatively affect us for the rest of our lives? That our ability to have intimate relationships, to trust, to digest physical or emotional experiences is forever and unalterably afflicted?

It was the opinion of my [Claudia's] guru, that there is always hope for change and healing. He told me "a doctor should always think that she will be able to find the goodness—she will be able to find the cure of the pain of the person." He didn't tell me there were certain conditions that were impossible to treat. He told me that the outcome of a treatment was not my concern. That was in the hands of God, but that it was our job, both as doctors and patients, to make the efforts.

So, what efforts might we make?

Gratefully, we have a loophole. If we apply our Law of Microcosm and Macrocosm to this dilemma, we see that we can use predawn through early morning as a window of opportunity to go back in time to change, heal and re-pattern early, stubborn, negative patterns, or to reinforce positive ones that were ingrained during our formative early life. Each new day ushers in a cascade of new possibilities and a shower of second chances. We can focus on pacifying Vata and encouraging the smooth flow of prana in these early morning hours.

Vata, by nature, is easily affected by influences—both positive and negative. Each morning we have a new opportunity to take advantage of this fact and engage in Vata-pacifying activities during these times.

If we follow the daily routine that the Ayurvedic sages recommend, we will be counteracting Vata's mobile, changeable qualities with the stability of routine. Since the sweet quality pacifies Vata, we can enjoy sweet sounds, fragrances, images, tastes, sensations and meditation.

The meditation and oil massages outlined in the daily routine both serve to pacify Vata and promote the smooth flow of prana. Additionally, notice that all the sense organs—the eyes, ears, nose, skin and mouth—are cleansed or oiled.

The first moments of a day set the tone for the day, as birth and the early days of an infant's life impact its lifetime. If we allow the first attention of the day to be peaceful, grateful and infused with a sense of joy, we are delivered into the new day as a healthy individual. And perhaps we are thereby healing the relative macrocosm of our in utero and birth experience at the same time, thereby benefiting our entire life.

Born Again in Radiance
Who can resist that first,
optimistic moment of dawn –
the dazzling sliver of light,
sun rising, rounding, making
the profound shift from
promise to presence.

*Every possibility contained
in a single instant; light
linking us to vastness,
light reaching back to the
formation of stars, light that
will not let us forget that we
are daily born again in radiance.*

Danna Faulds[4]

CHAPTER SUMMARY

Ayurveda works first with the physical, but its primary goal is the mind. It is the effects of Rajas and Tamas on the mind that create the disruption and distortion that can lead to addiction and disease. In a world filled with Rajasic stimulation and dysfunctional interactions, recovery beyond simple abstinence requires intentional effort to cultivate Sattva and re-establish a natural equilibrium that can flourish in new, unfolding ways and lead to true fulfillment and serenity. The promise of Ayurveda lies in daily renewal of our remembrance of our true nature.

SUGGESTED PRACTICE
Oil Ears with Warm Oil[5]

While some people enjoy filling each ear with about ten drops of warm oil and leaving it in each side for about ten minutes, others are more comfortable simply moistening the pinky finger with warm, untoasted sesame oil and lubricating the inside of the ear with this. Vata collects in empty spaces in the body and has a particular affinity with the ears and the sense of hearing, so this practice can help to pacify Vata, especially in the ears. It can be effective at helping ear diseases that are due to increased Vata, like some forms of tinnitus and loss of hearing, as well as for benefitting tissues and conditions in near proximity to the ears, stiff necks and temporomandibular joint.

Student Story—The Art of Living

It must be true when they say that "when you are ready, the teacher appears." My best friend told me about Yoga of Recovery in 2017, when I had initially stopped drinking and was searching for a rehab solution.

Learning YoR with Durga has shown me that becoming healthy is a long process. Just as addiction is progressive, the recovery is ongoing. Yoga, combined with studying Ayurveda principles, has opened up a world of healing and wholeness. But it also requires action and work toward those goals. While I have not relapsed with alcohol, it's all too easy to fall back into a poor mindset and to self-medicate with unhealthy foods and bad habits. Durga's teachings outline new ways of defining addictions in the context of everyday life. YoR instructs us in the art of living.

Myra W.

Student Story—Human Community

Yoga of Recovery has become a welcomed experiential learning gift to my recovery and life. With 33 years sober in 12-Step programs when I came to YoR, I had recovery processes that were well established—and YoR created a powerful community and path that deepened that healing yet again. I connected with people from all over the world, with contexts very different from each other, yet we all strongly identified with the framing of the teachings, as humans.

Doug R.

ENDNOTES

1   https://chopracentermeditation.com
2   For various information on ACEs see www.cdc.gov/violenceprevention/aces/index.html
3   Welch, *Dinacaryā*.
4   Faulds, D. (2002) 'Born Again in Radiance', in *Go In and In: Poems from the Heart of Yoga.* Greenville, VA: Peaceable Kingdom Books.
5   Welch, *Dinacaryā*.

Resources

Please visit my website www.yogaofrecovery.com for up-to-date links and suggestions on where to purchase the products you will need for some of the daily routines.

For many years, my main source has been **Banyan Botanicals** (USA). My practitioner page, showing my most-used products on their website, is www.banyanbotanicals.com/shop/practitioner/durga-leela.

I also recommend **Organic India** (USA; https://organicindiausa.com) and Pukka Herbs (UK; https://www.pukkaherbs.com/uk/en). These companies provide organic, fairly traded and sustainably sourced herbs from a network of farms in India and Sri Lanka.

For books and other yoga mat prop/wellness items, yoga teachers can buy in bulk with a great discount at **Integral Yoga Distribution** (https://new.iydistribution.com).

Gunas questionnaire

Diet:	☐ Vegetarian	☐ Some meat	☐ Heavy meat diet
Junk food/fast food:	☐ Never	☐ Occasionally	☐ Frequently
Caffeine/coffee, chocolate, sugar:	☐ Never	☐ Occasionally	☐ Frequently
Alcohol:	☐ Never	☐ Occasionally	☐ Frequently
Non-prescribed drugs:	☐ Never	☐ Occasionally	☐ Frequently
Prescription medications:	☐ Never	☐ As prescribed	☐ More frequently
Sensory impressions:	☐ Calm, pure	☐ Mixed	☐ Disturbed
Need for sleep:	☐ Little	☐ Moderate	☐ High
Sexual activity:	☐ Low	☐ Moderate	☐ High
Control of senses:	☐ Good	☐ Moderate	☐ Weak
Speech:	☐ Calm and peaceful	☐ Agitated	☐ Dull
Cleanliness:	☐ High	☐ Moderate	☐ Low
Work:	☐ Selfless	☐ For personal goals	☐ Lazy
Anger:	☐ Rarely	☐ Sometimes	☐ Frequently
Fear:	☐ Rarely	☐ Sometimes	☐ Frequently
Desire:	☐ Little	☐ Frequent	☐ Excessive
Pride:	☐ Modest	☐ Some ego	☐ Vain
Depression:	☐ Never	☐ Sometimes	☐ Frequently
Love:	☐ Universal	☐ Personal	☐ Lacking in love

Violent behavior:	☐ Never	☐ Sometimes	☐ Frequently
Attachment to money:	☐ Little	☐ Some	☐ A lot
Contentment:	☐ Usually	☐ Partly	☐ Never
Forgiveness:	☐ Easily	☐ With effort	☐ Holds grudges
Concentration:	☐ Good	☐ Moderate	☐ Poor
Memory:	☐ Good	☐ Moderate	☐ Poor
Willpower:	☐ Strong	☐ Variable	☐ Weak
Truthfulness:	☐ Always	☐ Most of the time	☐ Rarely
Honesty:	☐ Always	☐ Most of the time	☐ Rarely
Peace of mind:	☐ Generally	☐ Partly	☐ Rarely
Creativity:	☐ High	☐ Moderate	☐ Low
Spiritual study:	☐ Daily	☐ Occasionally	☐ Never
Mantra, prayer:	☐ Daily	☐ Occasionally	☐ Never
Meditation:	☐ Daily	☐ Occasionally	☐ Never
Service:	☐ Much	☐ Some	☐ None
Total:	Sattva	Rajas	Tamas ....

Ayurvedic constitutional assessment

Circle the descriptions that most apply to your long-term patterns. Give one point for each category. If descriptions from two columns apply, give half a point for each.

Category	Vata	Pitta	Kapha
Frame	Tall or short, thin, poorly developed physique	Medium, moderately developed physique	Stout, stocky, short, big, well developed physique
Weight	Low, hard to hold weight, prominent bones and veins	Moderate, good muscles	Heavy, tends toward obesity
Complexion	Dull, dark, brownish	Red, ruddy, flushed, glowing	White, pale
Skin texture	Thin, dry, rough, cracked, prominent veins	Moist, pink, with moles, freckles, acne	Thick, white, moist, soft, smooth
Temperature	Tends to feel cold	Tends to feel warm	Tends to feel cool
Hair	Scanty, coarse, dry, brown, slightly wavy	Moderate, fine, soft, early gray or bald	Abundant, oily, thick, very wavy, lustrous
Head	Small, thin, long, unsteady	Moderate	Large, stocky, steady
Forehead	Small, wrinkled	Moderate, with folds	Large, broad
Face	Thin, small, long, wrinkled, dusky, dull	Moderate, ruddy, sharp contours	Large, round, fat, white or pale, soft contours
Neck	Thin, long	Medium	Large, thick

Category	Vata	Pitta	Kapha
Eyebrows	Small, thin, unsteady	Moderate, fine	Thick, bushy, many hairs
Eyelashes	Small, dry, firm	Small, thin, fine	Large, thick, oily, firm
Eyes	Small, dry, thin, brown, dull, unsteady	Medium, thin, red (inflamed easily), green, piercing (deep-set)	Wide, prominent, thick, oily, white, attractive
Nose	Thin, small, long, dry, crooked	Medium, sharp (pointed)	Thick, big, firm, oily
Lips	Thin, small, darkish, dry, unsteady	Medium, soft, red	Thick, large, oily, smooth, firm
Teeth and gums	Thin, dry, small, rough, crooked, receding gums	Medium, soft, pink, gums bleed easily	Large, thick, soft, pink, oily
Shoulders	Thin, small, flat, hunched	Medium	Broad, thick, firm, oily
Chest	Thin, small, narrow, poorly developed	Medium	Broad, large, well or overly developed
Arms	Thin, overly small or long, poorly developed	Medium	Large, thick, round, well developed
Hands	Long, thin, dry, cold, rough, fissured, unsteady	Medium, warm, pink	Large, thick, oily, cool, firm
Thighs	Thin, narrow	Medium	Well developed, round, fat
Legs	Thin, excessively long or short, prominent knees	Medium	Large, stocky
Calves	Small, hard, tight	Loose, soft	Shapely, firm
Feet	Small, thin, long, dry, rough, fissured, unsteady	Medium, soft, pink	Large, thick, hard, firm
Joints	Small, thin, dry, unsteady, cracking	Medium, soft, loose	Large, thick, well built
Nails	Small, thin, dry, rough, fissured, cracked, darkish	Medium, soft, pink	Large, thick, smooth, white, firm, oily
Urine	Scanty, difficult, colorless	Profuse, yellow, red, burning	Moderate, whitish, milky

Feces	Scanty, dry, hard, difficult or painful, gas, constipation	Abundant, loose, yellowish, diarrhea, with burning sensation	Moderate, solid, sometimes pale in color, mucous in stool
Sweat/body odor	Scanty, no smell	Profuse, hot, strong smell	Moderate, cold, pleasant smell
Appetite	Variable, erratic	Strong, sharp	Constant, low
Taste preferences	Prefers sweet, sour or salty food, cooked with oil and spiced	Prefers sweet, bitter or astringent food, raw, lightly cooked without spices	Prefers pungent, bitter or astringent food, cooked with spices but not oil
Circulation	Poor, variable, erratic	Good, warm	Good, slow, steady
Activity	Quick, fast, unsteady, erratic, hyperactive	Medium, motivated, purposeful, goal-seeking	Slow, steady, stately, strong
Strength/ endurance	Low, poor endurance, starts and stops quickly	Medium, intolerant of heat	Endurance, but slow in starting
Sexual nature	Variable, erratic, deviant, strong desire but low energy, few children	Moderate, passionate, quarrelsome, dominating	Low but constant sexual desire, good sexual energy, devoted, many children
Sensitivity	Fear of cold/wind, sensitive to dryness	Fear of heat, dislike of sun/fire	Fear of cold/damp, likes wind and sun
Resistance to disease	Poor, variable, weak immune system	Medium, prone to infection	Good, prone to congestive disorders
Reaction to medications	Quick, low dosage needed, unexpected side effects or nervous reactions	Medium, average dosage	Slow, high dosage required, effects slow to manifest
Disease tendency	Nervous system diseases, pain, arthritis, mental disorder	Fevers, infections, inflammatory diseases	Respiratory system diseases, mucous, edema
Voice	Low, weak, hoarse	High pitched, sharp, moderate	Pleasant, deep, good tone
Speech	Quick, inconsistent, erratic, talkative	Moderate, argumentative, convincing	Slow, definite, not talkative

Category	Vata	Pitta	Kapha
Mental nature	Quick, adaptable, indecisive	Intelligent, penetrating, critical	Slow, steady, dull
Memory	Poor, notices things easily but forgets easily	Sharp, clear	Slow to take notice but will not forget
Finances	Earns and spends quickly, erratically	Spends on specific goals, causes or projects	Holds on to what's earned, particularly property
Emotional tendencies	Fearful, anxious, nervous	Angry, irritable, contentious	Calm, content, attached, sentimental
Neurotic tendencies	Hysteria, trembling, anxiety attacks	Extreme temper, rage, tantrums	Depression, unresponsiveness, sorrow
Faith	Erratic, changeable, rebel	Determined, fanatic, leader	Constant, loyal, conservative
Sleep	Light, tends toward insomnia	Moderate, may wake up but will fall asleep again	Heavy, difficulty in waking up
Dreams	Flying, moving, restless, nightmares	Colorful, passionate, conflict	Romantic, sentimental, watery, few dreams
Habits	Like speed, traveling, parks, plays, jokes, stories, trivia, artistic activities, dancing	Likes competitive sports, debates, politics, hunting, research	Likes water, sailing, flowers, cosmetics, business ventures, cooking
Total (50)			

Ayurvedic constitutional assessment courtesy of *Ayurvedic Healing* by Dr David Frawley